Springer Series on Medical Education

Carole J. Bland, PhD, Series Editor
Steven Jones, MD, Founding Editor

ABOUT THE EDITOR-IN-CHIEF

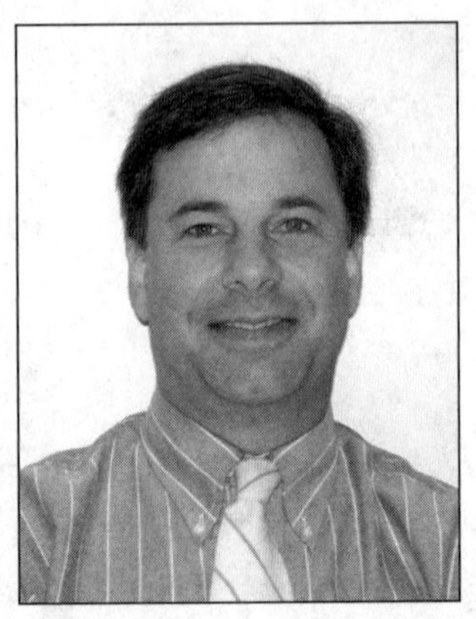 **Henry (Hank) Bernstein, D.O.** is an Associate Professor of Pediatrics at Harvard Medical School and Associate Chief of General Pediatrics at Children's Hospital Boston. He is board certified in Pediatrics and a Fellow of the American Academy of Pediatrics with more than twenty years of clinical experience as a primary care pediatrician in a variety of settings. In addition to his many administrative, teaching, and care responsibilities at Children's, he leads several national initiatives in medical education and clinical primary care research. Dr. Bernstein's interests focus on issues important to the community-based practice of primary care including health promotion, preventive health services, medical education, technology, postpartum newborn discharge, and clinical immunization development, education, and delivery. He has pioneered the development of several new and innovative teaching tools and other health promotion resources for both families and maternal and child health professionals.

Dr. Bernstein has been married to his wife Sophie for 25 years and has two beautiful children, 20-year-old Lauren and 14-year-old David.

Pediatrics in Practice

A Health Promotion Curriculum for Child Health Professionals

Henry H. Bernstein, DO

Editor-in-Chief

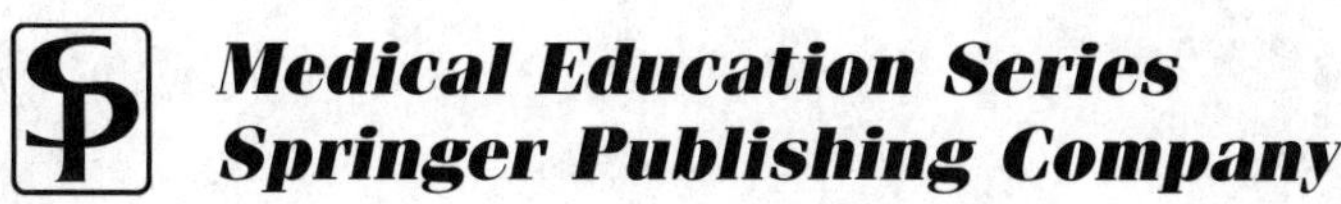

Medical Education Series
Springer Publishing Company

Springer Publishing Company, Inc.
11 West 42nd St.
New York, NY 10036-8002

Acquisitions Editor: Sheri W. Sussman
Production Editor: Jeanne W. Libby
Cover design by Joanne Honigman

Library of Congress Cataloging-in-Publication Data

Pediatrics in practice : a health promotion curriculum for child health professionals /
  Henry H. Bernstein, editor.
    p.   ; cm. — (Springer series on medical education)
  Includes bibliographical references and index.
  ISBN 0-8261-2725-8 (soft cover)
  1. Pedatrics—Study and teaching. 2. Health promotion.
  [DNLM: 1. Pediatrics—education. 2. Professional Practice.   WS 21 P3714 2005)   I.
Bernstein, Henry H. II. Series: Springer series on medical education (Unnumbered)

  RJ80.P43 2005
  618.92—dc22   2005007223

05 06 07 08/5 4 3 2 1

This book is dedicated to my wife Sophie, our children Lauren and David,
and my parents, Jeanette and the late Bernard Bernstein,
who have always been there for me with never-ending love, support,
and understanding.

It is our hope that the health and well-being of all children,
their families, and the communities where they live
are enhanced by the teachings in this curriculum.

Henry H. Bernstein, DO

CONTENTS

CONTRIBUTORS

Authors

John T. Benjamin, M.D.*
Chief, Division of Community Pediatrics
Professor of Pediatrics
The University of North Carolina at Chapel
  Hill
Chapel Hill, NC

Gregory S. Blaschke, M.D., M.P.H.* **
Program Director Pediatrics
Naval Medical Center San Diego
Assistant Professor of Pediatrics
University of California
San Diego, CA
Uniformed Services University of the Health
  Sciences
Bethesda, MD

Kara M. Connors, M.P.H.
Education Consultant
Division of General Pediatrics
Children's Hospital
Boston, MA

Donna M. D'Alessandro, M.D.*
Associate Professor of Pediatrics
Children's Hospital of Iowa
Roy J. and Lucille A. Carver College of Medi-
  cine
University of Iowa
Iowa City, IA

Janet Palmer Hafler, Ed.D.*
Assistant Professor of Medicine (Pediatrics)
Harvard Medical School Director of Faculty
  Development
Faculty Development Unit
Office of Educational Development
Harvard Medical School
Boston, MA

Danielle Laraque, M.D.*
Chief, Division of Pediatrics
Debra & Leon Black Professor of Pediatrics
Associate Professor of Pediatrics
Mount Sinai School of Medicine
New York, NY

Joseph O. Lopreiato, M.D., M.P.H.* **
Associate Professor of Pediatrics
Uniformed Services University of the Health
  Sciences
Bethesda, MD

Judith S. Palfrey, M.D.*
Chief, Division of General Pediatrics
Children's Hospital
T. Berry Brazelton Professor of Pediatrics
Harvard Medical School
Professor of Maternal and Child Health
Harvard School of Public Health
Boston, MA

Richard Pan, M.D., M.P.H.*
Associate Residency Director
Assistant Professor of Pediatrics
Department of Pediatrics
University of California, Davis
Sacramento, CA

Diane Pickles, B.A.*
Parent Consultant
Boston, MA

Emily J. Roth, M.D.
Instructor in Medicine
Harvard Medical School
Children's Hospital
Boston, MA

Theodore C. Sectish, M.D.*
Assistant Professor of Pediatrics
Stanford University School of Medicine
Residency and Clerkship Director
Packard Children's Hospital
  at Stanford University
Palo Alto, CA

Habib Shariat, M.D.*
Director, Ambulatory Pediatrics
Department of Pediatrics and Child Health
Howard University Hospital
Washington, DC

Judith S. Shaw, R.N., M.P.H.*
Nurse Consultant
Director, Vermont Child Health Improvement
  Program
Research Assistant Professor of Pediatrics
University of Vermont, College of Medicine
Burlington, VT

Franklin Trimm, M.D.*
Professor and Vice Chair of Pediatrics
Division of General Pediatrics
Director, Pediatric Residency Program
University of South Alabama Children's and
  Women's Hospital
Mobile, AL

Contributing Editors

Maria Alejandra Blanco, M.Ed.
Catherine Bodkin, LCSW, MSHA*
Marisa Brett, M.D.
Eugena Chan, M.D.
Sabrina Cimino, B.A.
Victoria Floriani, B.A.
Robert Heroux, B.A.
Sharon Levy, M.D.
Joshua Nagler, M.D.
Sarah Rieber, B.A.
Lori Rutman, B.A.
Rebecca Stoltz, B.A.
Ildiko Szabo

Technology Consultants

Video produced by:
Arlyn Bonfield, M.S.
Biomedical Media, Sharon, MA

Web site produced by:
Biomedical Media, Sharon, MA
     in collaboration with
Illumina Interactive, Boston, MA

Contributors/Evaluators

Michael Sesling
Kristen Breslin, M.D.
Mike Cotter, M.D.
Christy Duncan, M.D.
Eric Fleegler, M.D.
Alla Gruman, M.D.
Susan Hayden, M.D.
Jennifer Hyde, M.D.
Kate Jin, M.D.
Sharon Levy, M.D.
Carey Lumeng, M.D.
Heather McLauchlan, M.D.
Lisa McQueen, M.D.
Jeff Meadows, M.D.
Emily Milliken, M.D.
Jackie Owusu, M.D.
Elissa Rottenberg, M.D.
Heidi Shaff, M.D.
Jeff Skolnik, M.D.
Jessica Smith, M.D.
Laura Thomas, M.D.
Sara Toomey, M.D.
Sarah Wingerter, M.D.
University of Massachusetts Medical School
  Standardized Patient Program Instructors
      Wendy Gammon
      Trish Aponte
      Ellen Arcuri
      Ashley Ayers
      Eileen Bouchard
      Chelsea Gammon
      Toby Goldstein
      Becca Houston
      Maura Matarese
      Carmen Melendez
      Donna Richardson
      Jackie Therieau

Collaborators

American Academy of Pediatrics

Boston Combined Residency Program
  in Pediatrics

The Bright Futures Center for Pediatric Education in Growth and Development, Behavior
  & Adolescent Health

Continuity Clinic at Stanford's Pediatric Residency Training Program, Division of General Pediatrics

Harlem Hospital Pediatric Resource Center,
  New York, NY

Health Resources and Services Administration

Maternal and Child Health Bureau

Medical College of Georgia, Section of General Pediatrics and Adolescent Medicine, Department of Pediatrics, Augusta, GA

Mount Sinai Division of General Pediatrics, New York, NY

Naval Medical Center San Diego

Pediatric Health Associates

University Children's Medical Group at the University of California, Davis, Department of Pediatrics

University of Iowa Pediatric Residency Training Program

University of South Alabama Children's and Women's Hospital, Pediatric Residency Program, Mobile, AL

Print Production Team

Health Communication Connection
Carol Adams Rivera, M.A., project manager
Jeanne Anastasi, M.A., *Bright Futures* editor
Eileen Clark, B.A., *Bright Futures* editor
Oliver Green, B.S., graphic designer
Cynthia Landeen, Ph.D., indexer
Beth Rosenfeld, B.A., proofreader

FOREWORD

Everyone who has tried to build something knows that you need the right tools to have a finished product that works. A screwdriver will not work like a hammer, and a hammer will not work like a pair of pliers. The same can be said for how we deliver health promotion and prevention messages to families. The right tools are imperative to produce the outcomes our patients and families deserve and the public has a right to expect.

Equally important to having the right tools, is learning to use them when we are most "teachable". Given what we know about the antecedents of disease and building the foundation of a healthy lifetime, health promotion and disease prevention must be part of every child health encounter, whether a well child exam, an illness-related visit, or follow-up of a child who was hurt while biking without a helmet. The development of counseling and intervention skills should begin as early as possible in medical and child health professional education and be honed throughout the professional lifetime.

Pediatrics in Practice—A Health Promotion Curriculum for Child Health Professionals will support those of us who are teachers of health promotion and prevention. First, this publication is presented in an easy to use format that addresses early learners. Second, it provides opportunities for active participation of the students. Active learning is much more likely to produce the behaviors we want from our child health professionals. Third, it addresses key skills and attributes that are needed for success such as clinician-partnerships, communication, health promotion/disease prevention, time management, education, and advocacy. And fourth, experts have produced the content.

As we move further into an era of evidence-based medicine and measurement of both educational and clinical outcomes, it is our shared vision that all children will have a medical home in a system where effective health promotion and disease prevention thrive. *Curriculum for Child Health Professionals*, through its emphasis on early acquisition of essential skills by child health professionals, adds significantly to our ability to create a "brighter future" for all of our children.

Modena Wilson, MD, FAAP
Director, Department of Committees and
 Sections
American Academy of Pediatrics

Thomas Tonniges, MD, FAAP
Director, Department of Community
 Pediatrics
American Academy of Pediatrics

INTRODUCTION

Health Care in Context

The dramatic changes taking place in today's health care environment and in our nation's communities present an increasingly complex set of challenges for child health educators and professionals. The shift in health care delivery from acute to ambulatory care settings, the emphasis on cost-containment practices, changing demographics, increased health disparities among diverse groups within our population, and greater accountability among health care institutions—all shape a new climate for the education and practice of child health professionals. Perhaps most important, because of societal, behavioral, and lifestyle concerns, our children face increased health risks that are, for the most part, preventable.

These current challenges have generated an urgent examination of both education and practice programs in the health professions. Pediatric training programs, for example, must create educational and training solutions that are aligned with and responsive to health care delivery systems and the needs of children, families, and their communities. In the last decade, a growing number of maternal and child health initiatives have emerged to improve education and training in pediatrics.

The Bright Futures Approach

Notable among these initiatives is Bright Futures (www.brightfutures.org), a health promotion/illness prevention initiative created in 1990 through the sponsorship of the Health Resources and Services Administration's Maternal and Child Health Bureau and the Health Care Financing Administration's Medicaid Bureau. The mission of Bright Futures is "to promote and improve the health, education, and well-being of infants, children, adolescents, families, and communities" through specific goals such as enhancing the knowledge, skills, and practices of both health professionals and families, fostering partnerships between them, and promoting optimal health outcomes. Critical to achieving these goals is the development of Bright Futures–based materials to support health professionals and families in meeting the health and developmental needs of children.

Families report that child health professionals have done an excellent job of treating acute illnesses but have been less responsive to the pervasive and daily risks experienced by children and their families in recent decades, such as violence and gun-related injuries, drug use, and obesity. Addressing these often-preventable risks is one of the most compelling reasons for integrating a Bright Futures approach within clinical education and practice. *Bright Futures: Guidelines for Health Supervision of Infants, Children, and Adolescents,* first published in 1994 and last updated in 2002, was developed to help child health professionals address the current developmental and behavioral health challenges of children, families, and their communities.

A Bright Futures perspective highlights the essential role of health professionals not only in preventing or treating illnesses but also in incorporating health promotion into clinical practice in a time-efficient manner. The Bright Futures Health Promotion Work Group, comprising pediatricians, educators, parents, and nurses, was formed in 1998 to develop a curriculum that would support child health professionals in their health promotion efforts.

The Pediatrics in Practice Curriculum

The overall purpose of *Pediatrics in Practice,* the innovative curriculum developed by the Bright Futures Health Promotion Work Group, is to support child health professionals in integrating health promotion into clinical practice effectively and efficiently, thereby enhancing the health and well-being of children and families.

Available in both print and online formats, the curriculum consists of an introductory module, Health, with an accompanying videotape, *Bright Futures: Health Supervision for Infants, Chil-*

dren, and Adolescents; six stand-alone modules that present the curriculum's core concepts; and a facilitator's guide.

Core Concepts

The curriculum is based on six core concepts that serve as the foundation for effective health encounters:

- Partnership
- Communication
- Health Promotion/Illness Prevention
- Time Management
- Education
- Advocacy

Forming the basis for the curriculum's individual modules, these six concepts provide the tools for building successful partnerships and promoting positive interactions among health professionals, children, and families during health encounters. By learning how to integrate these core concepts into clinical practice, health professionals can be assured that they are delivering time-efficient health promotion services.

The underlying tenet of *Pediatrics in Practice* is that these core concepts can effectively guide clinical practice to enhance patient care. This curriculum helps child health professionals translate the core concepts into applied skills or competencies that build upon and enhance one another. Child health professionals with effective communication skills, for example, foster the development of health partnerships with the children and families they serve.

Finally, applying the core concepts of the curriculum in pediatric education and training programs fosters the advancement of competency requirements established by the Accreditation Council for Graduate Medical Education and other disciplinary associations in the areas of patient care, communication, professionalism, partnership-building, and work with diverse populations.

Curriculum Support for Educators

Expanding curricular opportunities that integrate health promotion content is only one strategy for improving health professional education and training. Faculty development is equally important. *Pediatrics in Practice* provides support for health professional educators in teaching health promotion content through a variety of learner-centered teaching strategies described in the curriculum's Facilitator's Guide.

The six key teaching strategies presented in the curriculum—case discussion, role-play, reflective exercise, brainstorming, buzz group, and mini-presentation—are used to convey health promotion content. These teaching strategies incorporate methods such as open-ended questions, active listening skills, and educational techniques like "teachable moments," which help educators model effective interactions between child health professionals and children and families.

Conclusion

Pediatrics in Practice teaches both the core concepts and the practical skills that support child health professionals in providing optimal care for children and their families in our complex and changing health care environment. This curriculum enables health professionals to form effective health partnerships and communicate through family- and child-centered messages; educate families through teachable moments and integrate health promotion in routine health encounters; identify and address each family's unique health concerns and needs in a time-efficient manner; and advocate for the health and well-being of families and the communities in which they live.

Kara M. Connors, M.P.H.
Henry H. Bernstein, D.O.

For More Information . . .

Pediatrics in Practice has been developed in both print and online format (www.pediatricsin practice.org). Additional information about the curriculum can also be found in Benjamin and colleagues (2002). If you have questions about the curriculum or how to use it, please contact:

Pediatrics in Practice
c/o Henry (Hank) Bernstein, D.O.
Children's Hospital
CHPCC, Hunnewell Ground
300 Longwood Avenue
Boston, MA 02115
Phone: (617) 355-7075
Fax: (617) 730-0505
E-mail:
pediatricsinpractice@childrens.harvard.edu

References

Bartlett, E.E., Grayson, M., & Barker R., et al. (1984). The effects of physician communication skills on patient satisfaction, recall, and adherence. *Journal of Chronic Diseases, 37,* 755–764.

Benjamin, J.T., Cimino, S.A., & Hafler, J.P., Bright Futures Health Promotion Work Group, & Bernstein, H.H. (2002). The office visit: A time to promote health—but how? *Contemporary Pediatrics, 19*(2), 90–107.

Green, M., & Palfrey, J.S., (Eds.) (2002). *Bright futures: guidelines for health supervision of infants, children, and adolescents* (2nd ed., rev.). Arlington, VA: National Center for Education in Maternal and Child Health.

Green, M., Palfrey, J.S., Clark, E.M., & Anastasi, J.M., (Eds.) (2002). *Bright futures: Guidelines for health supervision of infants, children, and adolescents* (2nd ed., rev.)—*Pocket guide.* Arlington, VA: National Center for Education in Maternal and Child Health.

Chapter 1

Facilitator's Guide

for

Pediatrics in Practice

Janet P. Hafler

CONTENTS

FACILITATOR'S GUIDE

OVERVIEW

In the context of children's developmental and behavioral health challenges, the ability to teach health promotion is a critical component of health professional education. Understanding how health promotion content is communicated to health professionals and then translated within various practice settings is essential. *Pediatrics in Practice* is a Bright Futures-based curriculum that provides the specific skills and strategies needed to teach health promotion and to foster a greater understanding of its core concepts among child health professionals.

Curriculum Components

Pediatrics in Practice: A Health Promotion Curriculum for Child Health Professionals consists of seven modules, presented in the following order:

1. *Health:* Introducing *Pediatrics in Practice* and Bright Futures (includes videotape)
2. *Partnership:* Building Effective Partnerships
3. *Communication:* Fostering Family-Centered Communication
4. *Health Promotion:* Promoting Health and Preventing Illness
5. *Time Management:* Managing Time for Health Promotion
6. *Education:* Educating Families Through Teachable Moments
7. *Advocacy:* Advocating for Children, Families, and Communities

Presenting the Modules

Format and Foundation Sessions

Each module contains either two or three sessions. Session 1 of each module represents the "foundation curriculum." Learners may complete the foundation curriculum to gain an understanding of the core concepts presented. Completion of the subsequent sessions within each module will provide topic enrichment of the concepts presented in the first session of each module.

Each module includes the following sections:

▶ **Overview**—synopsis of the module includes background, overall goal and objectives, instructional design with capsule description of sessions, teaching strategies, evaluation, guiding questions

▶ **Introduction to Teaching Sessions**—objectives for facilitator, materials needed (handouts, including evaluation forms; teaching aids), time allotted

▶ **Teaching Sessions**—step-by-step guidance in facilitating the session and enhancing learner participation (including a script for facilitators)

- Session Introduction (Bright Futures context, session objectives, guiding questions)
- Discussion and Exercises (primary material to be covered in the session)
- Take-Home Message
  - Answers to the Guiding Questions
  - Planning for the Next Session (optional)
  - Evaluation
- Handouts (including Session Evaluation Forms and Facilitator Self-Assessment Forms) are located at the end of each session

▶ **References and Resources**

Session Lengths and Settings

The teaching and application of the curriculum are appropriate in a variety of settings, from classroom to clinic. Within each module, the sessions can be presented individually as stand-alone sessions, or combined in an extended session. Although each session is designed to last approximately 30 minutes, the time suggested is a guideline to assist facilitators in planning. You may wish to consider unique variables that could influence the desired length of the session, and modify your teaching accordingly. (For example, with a large group of learners, you might consider modifying the introductions, which could potentially affect the length of the session.)

Components within the curriculum can be modified and adapted based on the learners' needs and experiences. For example, case vignettes are presented throughout the curriculum to highlight particular health concerns encountered by children and families. Educators utilizing the curriculum may wish to adapt the case vignettes to reflect the situations experienced by their learners and the children and families they work with. Similarly, reflective exercise questions may be expanded or adapted to respond to the particular learning styles or needs of the learners.

Evaluation and Assessment

To enhance both learning and teaching, the curriculum includes a **Session Evaluation Form** following each teaching session. Session Evaluation Forms provide opportunities for learners to evaluate the content and facilitation of the session and to offer additional comments and suggestions. (If teaching sessions are combined, use your discretion as facilitators in providing one evaluation form for multiple sessions within the module.)

A **Facilitator Self-Assessment Form** is also provided at the end of each session. As facilitators, you are encouraged to complete this form before and after each teaching experience (e.g., a single session or an entire module). This will allow you to assess your performance as a facilitator over time. (To view the evaluation and facilitation forms that follow each teaching session, please see the examples at the end of this guide.)

Using the Facilitator's Guide

The purpose of the Facilitator's Guide is to support health professional educators in gaining the knowledge, skills, and attitudes to teach health promotion content effectively. The guide is designed to enhance the implementation of the *Pediatrics in Practice* curriculum through a variety of learner-centered teaching strategies. These strategies include case discussion, role-play, reflective exercise, brainstorming, buzz group, and mini-presentation. While each teaching strategy presents certain benefits and challenges, this guide offers useful tips and step-by-step instructions to optimize the teaching experience.

Each module includes a script that the facilitator (designated by the icon ★) can use to introduce issues, ask reflective questions, prompt discussion, elicit feedback, and summarize important take-home messages. The script can be read or preferably paraphrased by the educator(s) facilitating the teaching sessions.

Intended for all skill levels, the Facilitator's Guide begins with a general overview of the facilitator's role and of ways to initiate the group learning process, such as making introductions and clarifying expectations. The guide then presents general teaching tips, information on fostering communication and providing feedback, overviews of the specific teaching strategies mentioned above, and a reference list.

PROMOTING A LEARNER-CENTERED APPROACH

Understanding Your Role As Facilitator

The facilitator guides the discovery of new ideas, knowledge, skills, and appropriate attitudes, and serves as a resource for learning. Skilled facilitation begins with understanding the needs of the learners and observing their interactions and behaviors. This enables the facilitator to play a major role in providing a safe and comfortable environment that fosters inclusiveness, openness, and sharing so that meaningful learning can occur. As facilitator, you can promote a rich learning environment by:

▶ Creating a climate that respects the learners' contributions and deters critical or judgmental attitudes

▶ Remaining neutral, without advancing your personal perspectives or ideas

- ▶ Asking clarifying questions that might suggest alternatives
- ▶ Keeping the group focused
- ▶ Encouraging participation

These key facilitative behaviors (Welch, 1999) form the basis for the Facilitator Self-Assessment Form that follows each session.

Introducing Your Group: Building a Relationship Between Facilitator and Learners

The process of group learning begins with introductions and with clarifying the roles and expectations of both the facilitator and the learners. These first interactions help build productive teaching/learning relationships. The following steps will help you introduce the learners to each other and establish a relaxed and receptive environment for the teaching session.

Welcoming the Learners to the Session

- ▶ Introduce yourself and invite the learners to do so also. Think of creative ways to handle introductions. For example, you could:
  - Let the learners know the name you prefer to be called, and ask them to indicate their own preference as they introduce themselves
  - Ask a question that invites them to respond about their past and current experiences
  - Elicit the learners' expectations for the session
- ▶ Communicate your goals and expectations relative to the topic and the class dynamic. Welcome the learners' contributions.
- ▶ Emphasize the need for active listening and respect.
- ▶ Reinforce your message through nonverbal behaviors in the following ways:
  - Maintain eye contact in your interactions
  - Move around the room during the session to engage all of the learners

- Listen attentively to each person's contributions
- Promote a supportive and relaxed environment

Setting the Context: The Bright Futures Concept

The World Health Organization has defined health as "a state of complete physical, mental and social well-being and not merely the absence of disease or infirmity." Bright Futures embraces this broad definition of health—one that includes not only prevention of morbidity and mortality, but also the achievement of a child's full potential. In the Bright Futures concept of health, providing the capacity for healthy child development is as important as ameliorating illness or injury. Recognizing and acknowledging the strengths and resources of the child, family, and community are essential to promoting healthy growth and development.

To build that capacity, the Pediatrics in Practice curriculum focuses on six core concepts: Partnership, Communication, Health Promotion/Illness Prevention, Time Management, Education, and Advocacy. The curriculum also includes a companion module (Health) and videotape that present an overview of Pediatrics in Practice and the Bright Futures approach.

Fostering Effective Communication

Promoting a learner-centered approach can help ensure the success of the teaching sessions. This can be achieved through informative and facilitative interventions. Heron (1989) developed a model of communication that can be used to analyze, guide, and develop skills in informative and facilitative interventions.

Informative Interventions

Informative interventions impart knowledge and interpret information in ways that enable learners to work from a more informed, resourceful position. You can achieve this by:

- ▶ Making instructions specific, behavioral, and measurable

- Limiting the amount of information given
- Giving the most important facts first
- Relating information clearly to the issue or problem being discussed
- Summarizing the information presented (carefully consider who should provide the end-of-session summary—you or one of the learners)

Facilitative Interventions

Facilitative interventions are designed to help learners become increasingly self-directed and reflective in their own learning. You can actively engage learners in their own learning by:

- Allowing them to reflect on their own experiences
- Encouraging them to raise, discuss, and answer their own questions
- Encouraging them to share ideas, and listening thoughtfully to the ideas expressed
- Allowing sufficient wait time (at least 3 seconds) when asking questions or probing ideas more deeply
- Promoting peer interaction

Providing Feedback

Feedback is fundamental to learning and/or improving skills. Feedback can reveal learners' strengths, identify areas needing improvement, and focus on ways to enhance learners' performance. Strategies for providing effective feedback include:

- Posing questions instead of giving direct answers.
- Providing feedback to the entire group, rather than to individuals. For example, in a case discussion, instead of offering positive feedback (e.g., Good question!) to one learner, generalize and redirect your response to all members of the group.
- Giving feedback according to the learners' needs by providing descriptive, specific, and positive feedback. This approach will foster a reservoir of goodwill, which helps learners become more receptive to constructive feedback.
- Asking learners to review their own performance and helping them evaluate their

performance in order to promote self-awareness and self-assessment. For example, you might ask, What do you believe are your strengths? What areas might need improvement? How would you develop a plan to address those areas?

USING SPECIFIC TEACHING STRATEGIES AND LEARNING FORMATS

The *Pediatrics in Practice* curriculum employs a number of learner-centered teaching strategies. These are listed below, followed by a brief overview of each strategy. One teaching strategy can be used to complement or enhance another. For example, a case discussion may incorporate role-play or reflective exercise. Case discussion is suggested as the core teaching strategy for this curriculum because each module is built around the learners' interaction with the content.

The teaching strategies used in the curriculum are:

1. Case Discussion
2. Role-Play
3. Reflective Exercise
4. Brainstorming
5. Buzz Group
6. Mini-Presentation

Case Discussion

Overview

Case discussion is used to develop analytic and problem-solving skills, and to explore solutions and various interpretations for complex reality-based issues. This teaching strategy can be especially helpful among learners with differing perspectives. Case discussion allows learners to develop and apply new knowledge and skills.

Applying the case discussion strategy requires reflective practice. Once a specific topic is mastered, the keys to effective case discussion are preparation and careful attention to content and group process.

Goals

The goals of case discussion as a teaching strategy are to:

▶ Develop critical-thinking skills.

▶ Provide opportunity for learners to use their knowledge in the discussion.

▶ Promote interactions among the learners.

Implementing the Strategy

Preparing to Present the Case

▶ Know the learners.

- In general, what level of knowledge and experience do they have?

- Address them by name, if possible.

- Meet the learners at their level. Encourage those at more advanced levels to teach others.

▶ Know your material.

- Review the goals for the case.

- Review the case, Facilitator's Guide, handouts, supplemental materials, and any references desired.

- If the case involves role-playing, select and prepare participants before beginning the discussion.

- Gather any additional materials you may need.

- Know the guiding questions for the case. Ask yourself, Why was this question suggested? Is its purpose to promote knowledge? Comprehension? Application? Analysis? Synthesis? Evaluation?

▶ Consider the various types of questions, and when/how you might use them. The role of the facilitator is to ask the right questions. Ask questions to keep the discussion going (answers typically interrupt the discussion).

- *Open-ended questions* promote learner-centered discussion (e.g., What are the major issues involved in this case?).

- *Closed questions* promote facilitator-centered discussion (e.g., What is the most important diagnostic finding in this case?).

- *Abstract questions* allow for a change in the direction of the discussion (e.g., How does this impact the patient's life?).

- *Challenge questions* make the discussion more specific (e.g., Why would that information help you?).

Introducing the Case

▶ Discuss the ground rules. This is a case discussion, not a lecture.

▶ Plan questions that shift the focus from you as facilitator to the learners. Remember that good questions sharpen critical thinking and serve as a model for learners to develop their own questions.

▶ Be prepared to let the discussion go in directions you did not intend (learner-centered discussion).

▶ Create a safe environment. Avoid calling on people directly but facilitate group interaction by summarizing a learner's remarks and relating them to ideas or questions contributed by other speakers.

▶ Be enthusiastic—it's contagious!

Beginning the Discussion

▶ Ask a volunteer to read the first part of the case or the entire vignette.

▶ Elicit a learning agenda for the case. Ask the learners what issues they see in the case, and write their responses on the display board or flip chart. Prioritize the issues and move into the discussion. This will give both the group and the facilitator a reference point and a list to review or summarize at the end of the case. Items not addressed can be included in handouts and/or reference readings, or can be pursued individually.

Facilitating the Discussion

▶ Summarize, analyze, and emphasize key points.

▶ Redirect questions asked of you (as facilitator) back to the group (e.g., "What do others think?").

▶ Refer to key points other learners have made.

▶ State or ask how what was said relates to the case.

▶ Remember that discussion is diminished when:

  • Factual questions are asked rapidly ("'What am I thinking?' game").

  • Learners' questions are immediately answered by the facilitator.

  • The wait time after asking questions is insufficient (waiting more than 3 seconds after a question is asked helps promote discussion).

  • Responses are judged (e.g., Good answer!).

▶ Remember that discussion is enhanced when the facilitator uses questions that focus on:

  • Diagnosis: What's going on?

  • Action: What would you do in this situation?

  • Information: How many? What happened?

  • Challenge: How do we know that?

  • Extension: How is that related to the case?

  • Priority: What is most important?

  • Prediction: What will happen next?

> Example:
>
> In Session 2 of the Partnership module (page 53), the facilitator uses a case vignette to lead the learners through a discussion that focuses on six essential steps for building effective partnerships with families. After the learners have read the case vignette, the facilitator reviews the six steps and poses questions for group discussion. For example, step 2 of the partnership-building model states the importance of identifying the health issues or concerns of families through interview questions and active listening.
>
> The facilitator generates discussion by asking the learners what issues the family has communicated in the vignette, and how they as health professionals might seek feedback and clarification on those issues. To achieve this goal, the facilitator asks, "What would you like to ask the mother?" The learners then respond with questions, which the facilitator lists on a display board. After a review of these questions, the facilitator summarizes the specific interview questions the child health professional might ask to determine the central issues facing the family.

  • Generalization: Can you think of other situations that may apply?

▶ Allow silences or sufficient wait time. This gives learners time to reflect on the question and respond.

▶ Be an active listener. Listen for:

  • Content of answers: facts, logic, intellectual information.

  • Continuity of answers: Who spoke? What was said? In what context? Were unspoken assumptions used when making statements?

  • Mechanics: body language, contributions mumbled versus spoken loudly.

  • Emotion: Are absolutes or conditionals used? Are emphatic statements made?

  • Listening ability: If this is absent, ask the learner to restate the question or statement before responding.

▶ Make brief statements to:
  • Declare a factual item.
  • Emphasize a principle by repeating it as stated.
  • Synthesize a concept by paraphrasing it in a different form.
  • Summarize key items.
▶ Redirect the discussion by reflecting the question or issue back to the group when …
  • Discussion is dominated by an individual.
  • Incorrect information is presented. Ask the person to explain the reasoning, or poll the other members of the group. You might ask, "Does everyone agree with that?"

Role-Play

Overview

In role-play, designated learners (or professional actors) assume a role, playing themselves or another person in a given situation or scenario, based on the objectives of the teaching session. Those involved in role-play are expected to "act out" the demands of the particular situation or role on their own or with a trained expert. Role-play situations may be reality-based or imaginative, and the scope of complexity may vary.

The role-play method provides the opportunity for learners to gain new knowledge and appreciate different points of view and perspectives, based on the role(s) being played. Role-play also helps learners develop and practice new skills and behaviors, such as improving communication, exploring solutions, and resolving conflict. Through the role-play method, educators are well-positioned to analyze the learners' reactions and responses, and peers can give direct and immediate feedback (Steinert, 1993).

Goal

The goal of role-play as a teaching strategy is to:
▶ Foster, and allow opportunities for practicing, new skills and behaviors.

Implementing the Strategy

Establishing Learner Goals

Ask one of the learners to read the case aloud at the beginning of the session, so that all are familiar with it (excluding features meant to be withheld from those assigned specific roles). The learners then generally discuss the case and identify learning goals for the exercise. Alternatively, some cases already include detailed learning goals. If so, the goals can still be discussed and adapted for the session's purposes. In establishing goals, learners might think in terms of what they would like to accomplish, how they would go about doing so, and how they would know whether the goal was accomplished.

Choosing Roles for Learners

Ask the learners to divide into small groups (typically groups of three, with each person playing a role). Practicing a role-play in a small group offers the opportunity for learners to feel safer than if practicing in front of the entire group. Some experienced facilitators advise selecting the individuals for each role at the beginning of the teaching session rather than immediately before starting the exercise. This removes the suspense of learners' worrying about whether they will be selected, instead of concentrating on the topic. Use this strategy only when the group members feel safe and comfortable with each other (which often requires about three meetings with the same group members).

Assigning Roles to Observers

To enhance the sense of participation by those who are not acting out a role, you might assign roles in observation and feedback. Ask learners to give feedback on a specific goal identified by one of the role-players in the case simulation. Alternatively, after listening to the discussion, ask whether learners would volunteer to give feedback related to their interests. For example, you might ask, "Would you give feedback on the nonverbal behavior?" It is usually best to assign roles early in the session to as many learners as possible.

Setting Up the Exercise

It is important that the group agree on how the exercise will be run. This includes deciding how long the case simulation will last, who

Example:

In Session 2 of the Education module (page 207), the facilitator introduces a role-play exercise to focus on the concept of wait time. The facilitator asks the learners to form groups of three, with each learner taking a turn playing the role of health professional ("teacher"), child, and father. Specific instructions are provided so learners can experience the importance of wait time. For example, the "teacher" is required to ask the father a series of questions, but must wait at least 3–5 seconds after each response before asking the next question. Following the exercise, the facilitator asks, "How did having to wait make you feel?" After the discussion, the facilitator concludes with feedback about the importance of incorporating wait time into conversations with families.

can interrupt, and whether others will take turns playing various roles. Being asked to role-play in front of a group is always more stressful than anticipated. If others will be asked to take turns playing roles, it is important to establish this ahead of time so the initial role-players don't feel they have been replaced because of a lackluster performance.

Giving Feedback

The classic sequence for giving feedback involves first asking the role-player(s) involved in the simulated case, "How did that go for you? What did you see happen, from your perspective? What would you like to have done differently?" Then open the process to the rest of the group.

Providing Learner-Centered Feedback

Learner-centered feedback is recommended because it allows the learners more control and focuses on their issues. In this feedback strategy, the facilitator continues to probe the experience by asking the learner, "Why did this work well? How might this have gone better for you? What would you like to have done differently?" and other similar questions. The learner's replies control the feedback, which becomes focused on the concrete issues of the interview. This method of providing feedback by interacting with the learners has proven more effective than giving a list of suggestions in the guise of feedback. Those who played specific roles have the opportunity at this time to discuss their role-play experience and what they learned from it.

Discussion and Analysis

The final segment should be devoted to a discussion of the learning goals for the exercise. The facilitator asks for feedback on the learning: "What did the learners learn? What, in particular, made this an effective learning exercise?" The emphasis on providing concrete, useful feedback that is learner centered will be recognized and appreciated by the learners. Those who played specific roles have the opportunity at this time to discuss their role-play experience and what they learned from it.

Reflective Exercise

Overview

A reflective exercise creates opportunities for individuals or groups to reflect on and examine their beliefs and practices related to an action or experience, gain a deeper understanding of the issue(s), and construct their own meaning and significance (Dewey, 1993, Moon, 1999). As part of the reflective exercise, the facilitator should provide clear directions to the learners and guide them through each step of the exercise.

Goals

The goals of reflective exercise as a teaching strategy are to:

▶ Engage learners in a continuous practice of self-observation and self-evaluation in order to understand their behavior and improve their practice.

▶ Motivate learners to advance from surface learning (e.g., rote memory) to deeper learning (e.g., interaction at a high level with content).

Implementing the Strategy

Reflective exercises are used to introduce learners to the benefits of reflecting on the learning process. Integrating reflective exercises into either a case discussion or didactic teaching (and other forms of teaching) empowers learners not only to recall what they have learned (rote memory) but also to "make sense" of it, form judgments about it, and modify it appropriately to enhance their expertise and practice (Moon, 1999). Common methods for fostering reflective practice are the use of journals and group discussion (in person or electronically).

Brainstorming

Overview

Brainstorming is a learning activity or technique to encourage the generation of creative ideas. Typically, brainstorming is a group process in which members contribute suggestions in a spontaneous, noncritical manner. The process often concludes with a summary of the ideas generated, with additional analysis or discussion. The facilitator may wish to identify certain patterns that have emerged from the list of ideas. Brainstorming is useful at all levels of problem-solving, from the initial attempt to formulate broad concepts to the final, detailed definition. (This group problem-solving method was given its name by Alexander Osborn, founding partner of the advertising firm Batten, Barten, Durstine, and Osborn [Osborn, 1957].)

Goal

The goals of brainstorming as a teaching strategy are to:

▶ Encourage each person to generate an idea.
▶ Begin developing a collaborative process of group work.
▶ Generate ideas that can set the stage for prioritizing ideas.

Implementing the Strategy

The facilitator convenes a group, typically 5–10 persons, to work on a specific question or issue, and asks the learners to spontaneously express whatever ideas comes to mind. The facilitator writes the ideas on the board legibly so everyone can read them, and encourages all learners to freely express their ideas to promote a respectful environment. Learners are asked not to criticize any of the ideas offered or to dominate the session. The facilitator then lists all suggestions, using the learners' words. Prioritizing the suggestions to identify patterns that emerge can be done at the end of the exercise.

Playing by the Rules

Although sessions can be guided by many rules, Osborn (1957) emphasizes the following:

▶ Never evaluate or judge a response. Judgmental attitudes may cause learners to be more concerned with defending ideas than generating them. This is probably the most important factor in brainstorming, which should allow great diversity in pooling opinions and ideas.

▶ Encourage learners to think of all possible ideas. Encouraging all ideas is more effective than limiting ideas to a particular focus. Osborn suggests that "combinations or modifications of previously suggested ideas often lead to new ideas that are superior to those that sparked them" (Adams, 1986, p. 136).

▶ Promote a *quantity* of ideas because quantity helps control the tendency toward

Example:

In the Advocacy module (page 228), the facilitator begins by asking the learners, "How would you define advocacy? When you hear the phrase 'to advocate' or the word 'advocacy,' what are some words that come to mind?" The facilitator lists the learners' responses, and, if necessary, prompts the group by providing some suggestions. After a number of ideas have been generated, the facilitator reviews the list, cites the *American Heritage Dictionary* definition of advocacy, and concludes with the observation that advocacy can be defined in many ways. The facilitator then begins to focus the discussion on advocacy in the context of the child's and family's health concerns.

"internal evaluation" and also leads to *quality*.

Buzz Group

Overview

Buzz groups offer an effective strategy for promoting small-group interactions among learners. In buzz groups, small numbers of learners work together around a particular focus or task. This teaching strategy can be integrated into lectures, case discussions, and presentations.

Goals

The goals of the buzz group as a teaching strategy are to:

▶ Foster collaboration.

▶ Increase participation among all members of the group.

Example:

In the Communication module (page 74), the buzz group format is used in conjunction with a reflective exercise and a videotaped segment from the film *The Doctor*. This segment illustrates the physician-centered communication style. Following a brief, uninterrupted reflective exercise, the facilitator convenes buzz groups by asking the learners to turn to the person next to them and to describe as fully as possible in the next 2 minutes their thoughts about the physician's communication skills as presented in the videotape. To guide discussion, the facilitator lists a series of questions on the board:

• What is your reaction to the video?

• What methods did the physician use to elicit the agenda of the patient?

• What aspects of the interview contributed to good/bad communication?

After discussion among the buzz groups, the facilitator then asks, "Who would like to describe their reflections?" This sets the stage for the learners to engage in discussion and to report back to the larger group.

- Activate learners' prior knowledge.
- Serve as a method for problem-solving.

Implementing the Strategy

Establishing the Buzz Group

Buzz groups can be assigned or can evolve naturally. A large group may be divided into smaller groups by the facilitator for a brief discussion on a given topic. Members of the buzz groups should introduce themselves unless all learners in the session know one another.

Buzz Group Format

Although buzz groups can have different formats, a typical format would involve a group of two or more persons discussing a question, problem, issue, or idea posed by the facilitator. (The facilitator may choose to write the question or idea under discussion on the board as a visual reminder.)

Members of the buzz group may be asked to develop hypotheses, solutions, or ideas they believe are relevant to the topic. The group should be given a specified time to work, typically ranging from 1 to 5 minutes, depending on the task. A buzz group leader may report back to the larger group, or volunteers from a few of the groups can share their ideas.

Mini-Presentation

Overview

Mini-presentations are an effective strategy for conveying information to learners in a brief period of time (typically 5 minutes or less). The information is presented in lecture format.

Goal

The goal of mini-presentation as a teaching strategy is to:

- Convey information that is not easily accessible in written formats.

Implementing the Strategy

The following tips help ensure effective presentations:

- Define your goals and make sure the content of the lecture is organized.

- Assess the learners' knowledge base and try to gauge their interest in the topic. Ask yourself, "How can I promote their interest in the presentation?"
- Think about your delivery skills (voice, eye contact, body movement, facial expressions). Could any of these skills benefit from additional attention or practice?
- Be prepared to use audiovisual materials such as slides, overhead transparencies, a chalkboard or display board, and videotapes. Arrive early to place, test, or prepare any materials or devices you plan to use.
- Integrate effective teaching strategies in your presentation. Ask yourself, "What applications for problem-solving or decision-making are included in the presentation? What opportunities for interaction with the learners could be built into the presentation?" Some strategies for increasing participation include convening an initial brainstorming session to identify possible questions; forming buzz groups to discuss the issue; or asking learners to "vote" on an issue at different points in the presentation or discussion.

Example:

In Session 1 of the Education module (page 192), the facilitator introduces a process for the learners to practice a mini-presentation. Learners are divided into groups to practice different teaching strategies. One of the groups is asked to use the "telling" strategy by developing a 1-minute presentation for family members on how to use a thermometer. The facilitator provides specific instructions, asking the group members to put themselves in the family's position and construct their presentation based on what they would need to know as family members. Each teaching group is given 10 minutes to complete the exercise based on a specific teaching strategy, and then present it to the entire group.

CONCLUDING THE TEACHING SESSION

The following key steps may be considered when concluding each teaching session:

▶ Summarize—or ask a learner to summarize—the main topics addressed in the session.

▶ Restate the articulated goals of the group.

▶ Review, highlight, and emphasize the take-home messages.

To enhance your own learning as a facilitator, think about the process of your teaching and facilitation:

▶ Reflect on the following (if applicable to the teaching strategy):

- Which questions worked for you?
- How well did they work?
- Did they accomplish the intended purpose in the discussion?

▶ Encourage learners' continued reflection by proposing self-learning approaches (e.g., keeping a journal) to deepen their understanding of the topic.

▶ Express your interest, as facilitator, in continuing to share the learners' progress or questions in addressing the core concepts.

Evaluation and Facilitation Forms

▶ Distribute the Session Evaluation Form(s) and collect the completed forms.

▶ Complete the Facilitator Self-Assessment Form.

[Module Name]: Session 1

SESSION EVALUATION FORM

Session 1: [Name of Session]

Date: _______________________

Facilitator(s): _______________________

Site: _______________________

1. Overall, I found the [session title] session to be:

Not Useful				Very Useful
1	2	3	4	5

2. The objectives of the session were:

Not Clear				Clear
1	2	3	4	5

3. The organization of the session was:

Poor				Excellent
1	2	3	4	5

4. The communication skills of the facilitator(s) were:

Poor				Excellent
1	2	3	4	5

5. The facilitator(s) stimulated interest in the subject matter:

Not at All				Very Much
1	2	3	4	5

6. The facilitator(s) encouraged group participation:

Not at All				Very Much
1	2	3	4	5

7. Handouts or visual aids (if used) were:

Not Helpful				Very Helpful
1	2	3	4	5

8. Any additional comments?

____
____
____

9. The most useful features of the session were:

____
____
____

10. Suggestions for improvement

____
____
____

11. Suggestions for topics related to this session

____
____
____

[Module Name]: Session 1

FACILITATOR SELF-ASSESSMENT FORM

Directions: Please rate yourself from 1 to 5 on the following facilitator skills. The closer you are to a 5 within each domain, the more skilled you are at facilitation. We encourage you to complete this form prior to and after each teaching experience (e.g., a single session or an entire module). This will allow you to assess your performance as a facilitator over time.

Facilitator Behavior	1	2	3	4	5
Remains neutral					
Does not judge ideas					
Keeps the group focused on common task					
Asks clarifying questions					
Creates a climate free of criticism					
Encourages participation					
Structures participation					

Source: Adapted with permission from Welch, M. (1999). *Teaching diversity and cultural competence in health care: A trainer's guide.* San Francisco, CA: Perspectives of Differences Diversity Training and Consultation for Health Professionals (PODSDT).

References

Adams, J.L. (1986). *Conceptual blockbusting*. Menlo Park, CA: Addison-Wesley Publishing Co.

Arseneau, R., & Rodenburg, D. (1998). The developmental perspective: Cultivating ways of thinking. In D.D. Pratt (Ed.), *Five perspectives on teaching in adult and higher education*. Malabar, FL: Kreigner Publishing.

Barnes, L., Christensen, C., & Hansen, A. (1994). *Instructor's guide to teaching and the case method* (3rd ed.). Boston: Harvard Business School Press.

Boud, D., Keough, R., & Walker, D. (Eds.) (1985). *Reflection: Turning experience into learning*. London: Kogan Page.

Coles, C., & Fish, D. (1997). *Developing professional judgement in health care*. Oxford, UK: Butterworth-Heinemann.

Dewey, J. (1993). *How we think: A restatement of the relation of reflective thinking to the educative process*. Boston: Houghton Mifflin Company.

Dillon, J.T. (1990). *The practice of questioning*. London: Routledge.

Ende, J. (1983). Feedback in clinical medical education. *JAMA, 250,* 777–781.

Heron, J. (1975). *Six category intervention analysis*. UK: University of Surrey, Human Potential Research Project.

Heron, J. (1989). *The facilitator's handbook*. London: Kogan Page.

Knight, J.R., & Emans, S.J. (Eds.) (2001). *Bright futures case studies for primary care clinicians: A guide to the case teaching method; and growth in children and adolescents*. Boston, MA: Bright Futures Center for Education in Child Growth and Development, Behavior and Adolescent Health. [Information on Case-Based Teaching available online at www.pedicases.org/teaching.phtml.]

Kroenke, K. (1984). The lecture: Where it wavers. *The American Journal of Medicine, 77,* 393–396.

Moon, J. (1999). *Reflection in learning and professional development*. London: Kogan Page Limited.

Napell, S. (1976). Six common non-facilitating teaching behaviors. *Contemporary Education, 47*(2), 199–202.

Osborn, A. (1957). *Applied imagination*. New York: Charles Scribner's Sons.

Osterman, K., & Kottham, R. (1993). *Reflective practice for educators: Improving schooling through professional development*. Newbury Park, CA: Corwin Press, Inc.

Pratt, D., & Magill, M.K. (1983). Educational contracts: A basis for effective clinical teaching. *Journal of Medical Education, 58,* 462–467.

Rogers, C., & Farson, R. (1955). *Active listening. seminar program for instructors in professional schools; Cases and readings*. Chicago: University of Chicago, Industrial Relations Center.

Rowe, M.B. (1986). Wait time: Slowing down may be a way of speeding up! *Journal of Teacher Education, 37,* 43–50.

Schmidt, H. (1983). The rationale behind problem-based learning. *Journal of Medical Education, 17,* 11–16.

Schön, D.A. (1983). *The reflective practitioner*. New York: Basic Books, Inc.

Schwenk, T.L., & Whitman, N. (1987). [Lectures.] In *The physician as teacher*. Baltimore, MD: Williams and Wilkins.

Simpson, M.A. (1985). How to use role-play in medical teaching. *Medical Teacher, 7,* 75–82.

Steinert, Y. (1993). Twelve tips for using role-plays in clinical teaching. *Medical Teacher, 15*(4), 283.

Tiberius, R.G. (1990). *Small group teaching*. Toronto: OISE Press/The Ontario Institute for Studies in Education Press.

Welsh, M. (1999). *Teaching diversity and cultural competence in health care: A trainer's guide*. San Francisco, CA: Perspectives of Differences Diversity Training and Consultation for Health Professionals (PODSDT).

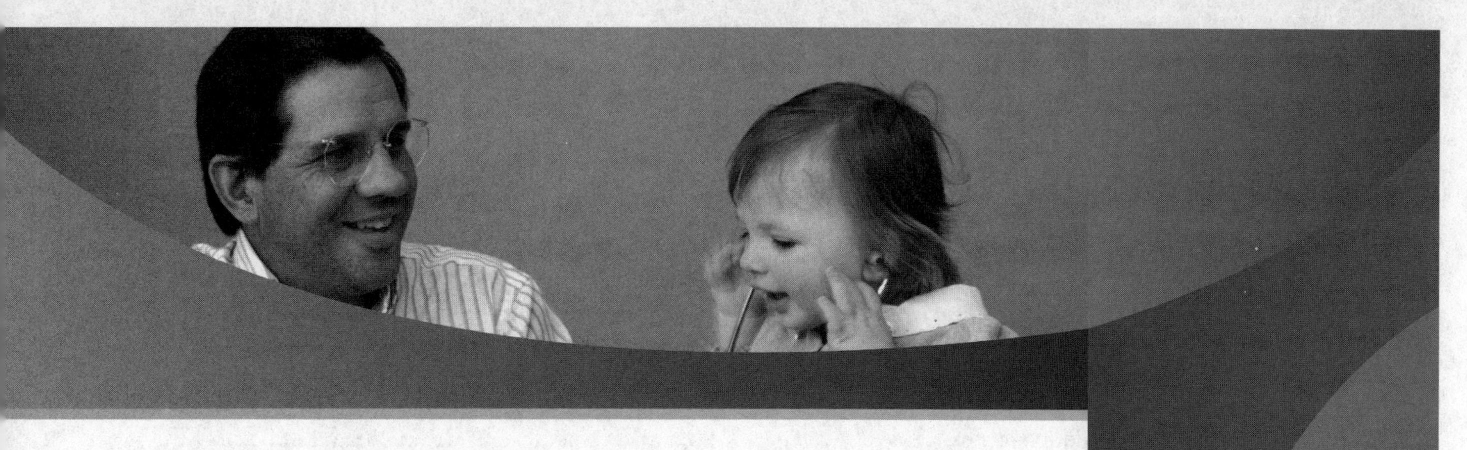

Health

Introducing Pediatrics in Practice and Bright Futures

Richard Pan

Habib Shariat

Judith S. Palfrey

CONTENTS

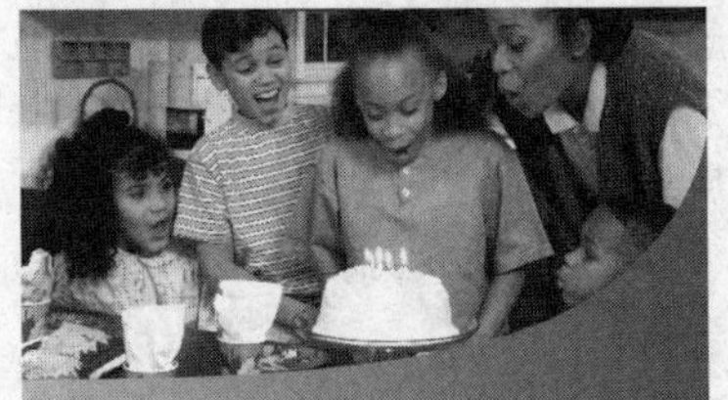

HEALTH
Introducing Pediatrics in Practice *and Bright Futures*

OVERVIEW

Background

Pediatrics in Practice is a health promotion curriculum based on Bright Futures, a child health initiative that invites child health professionals to adopt a broad definition of health—one that goes beyond the absence of illness or infirmity. *Pediatrics in Practice* seeks to enhance child health professionals' knowledge, skills, and practice to ensure that our nation's children and adolescents can lead happy, healthy lives and reach their full potential—physically, mentally, emotionally, and socially—to become responsible adults and contributing members of the community. Bright Futures recognizes that child health professionals, families, and communities need to work together to achieve this goal.

Goal

The overall goal of this module is to help learners broaden their understanding of health beyond the mere absence of illness or infirmity, and to introduce six core concepts based on Bright Futures content and philosophy: Partnership, Communication, Health Promotion/Illness Prevention, Time Management, Education, and Advocacy.

This module will enable learners to:

▶ Explore and expand their definition and understanding of the "healthy child"

▶ Understand the six core concepts addressed in the *Pediatrics in Practice* curriculum

▶ Gain a greater awareness of how children's health depends on the health of their families and communities

▶ Understand the importance of acknowledging the strengths of the child, family, and community as partners in health

▶ Identify the child's, family's, and health professional's concerns or agendas during a health visit

▶ Recognize the health professional's role in supporting families and communities in promoting children's health

Instructional Design

This module consists of two 30-minute sessions.

▶ Session 1 presents an overview of health, introduces the *Pediatrics in Practice* core concepts, and incorporates the videotape *Bright Futures: Health Supervision of Infants, Children, and Adolescents.*

▶ Session 2 presents an in-depth look at effective strategies that pediatric providers can use to help children achieve optimal health.

▶ Each of the two sessions can be used as a separate, stand-alone offering, or the sessions can be combined. See the Facilitator's Guide for information on combining sessions.

Teaching Strategies

The teaching strategies used in this module include case discussion, reflective exercise, and brainstorming. These strategies have been selected to help learners develop the skills required to promote optimal health among children and their families. Please refer to the Facilitator's Guide for more information related to each strategy.

Evaluation

The Health module serves primarily as an introduction to the six other *Pediatrics in Practice* modules, each with its own evaluation component. Learners will complete a **Session**

Evaluation Form following each session. Facilitators are encouraged to complete a **Facilitator Self-Assessment Form** prior to and following each teaching experience (e.g., a single session or an entire module) in order to assess their performance over time.

Guiding Questions

Learners who have completed the entire Health module should be able to answer the following questions:

▶ What is a "healthy" child in the context of the family and community?

▶ What are the six core concepts that support Bright Futures?

▶ How do I, as a pediatric provider, identify the strengths of a child, family, and community?

▶ How do I identify which concerns or agendas should be addressed during a health visit?

Reflecting on Your Practice

At the end of any clinical session, facilitators or clinical preceptors may engage learners in the following reflective questions. These questions are designed to promote critical thinking related to practice change.

▶ At which health visits today did you identify a specific strength or achievement of the family, and affirm or acknowledge it during the visit?

▶ At which health visits today did you identify the child's and the family's primary concerns or agendas for the visit?

INTRODUCTION TO TEACHING SESSIONS

Session 1: Health and the Bright Futures Concept

Objectives

The objectives for this session are for the facilitator to:

▶ Help learners explore and expand their definition and understanding of the "healthy child"

▶ Introduce the six core concepts addressed in the *Pediatrics in Practice* curriculum: Partnership, Communication, Health Promotion/Illness Prevention, Time Management, Education, and Advocacy

▶ Foster a greater awareness of how children's health depends on the health of their families and communities

Materials

The materials and teaching aids needed for this session are:

Handouts

▶ Bright Futures Children's Health Charter

▶ Session Evaluation Form

Facilitator Form

▶ Facilitator Self-Assessment Form

Teaching Aids

▶ Videotape *Bright Futures: Health Supervision of Infants, Children, and Adolescents*

▶ VCR and monitor

▶ Display board, flip chart, or chalkboard

▶ Markers or chalk

▶ 8 1/2" x 11" paper

Time

The time allocated for this session is 30 minutes.

Session 2: Just Another Healthy Child?

Objectives

The objectives for this session are for the facilitator to:

▶ Emphasize the importance of acknowledging the strengths of the child, family, and community as partners in health

▶ Help learners identify the child's, family's, and health professional's concerns or agendas during a health visit

▶ Foster recognition of the health professional's role in supporting families and communities in promoting children's health

Materials

The materials and teaching aids needed for this session are:

Handouts
▶ Case Vignette: Janice's 10 Year Visit
▶ Bright Futures Interview Questions for 10 Year Visit
▶ Case Growth Chart
▶ Session Evaluation Form

Facilitator Form
▶ Facilitator Self-Assessment Form

Teaching Aids
▶ Display board, flip chart, or chalkboard
▶ Markers or chalk

Time

The time allocated for this session is 30 minutes.

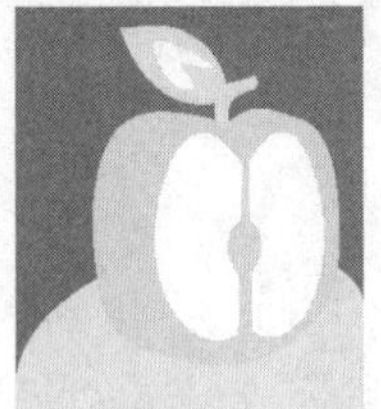

SESSION 1:

Health and the Bright Futures Concept

At the beginning of the session, the facilitator and learners should introduce themselves briefly. Ideas for creative introductions can be found in the Facilitator's Guide.

Setting the Context: The Bright Futures Concept

The facilitator **(F)** introduces the learners to the Bright Futures concept of health by reading or paraphrasing the following:

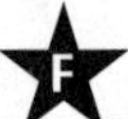

The World Health Organization has defined health as "a state of complete physical, mental and social well-being and not merely the absence of disease or infirmity." Bright Futures embraces this broad definition of health—one that includes not only prevention of morbidity and mortality, but also the achievement of a child's full potential. In the Bright Futures concept of health, providing the capacity for healthy child development is as important as ameliorating illness or injury. Recognizing and acknowledging the strengths and resources of the child, family, and community are essential to promoting healthy growth and development.

To build that capacity, the Pediatrics in Practice *curriculum focuses on six core concepts: Partnership, Communication, Health Promotion/Illness Prevention, Time Management, Education, and Advocacy. The curriculum also includes a companion module (Health) and videotape that present an overview of* Pediatrics in Practice *and the Bright Futures approach.*

Introducing the Session

Before introducing the session, the facilitator distributes the handout **Bright Futures Children's Health Charter.**

Note to facilitator: Learners should be chal-lenged throughout the discussion to broaden their definition and deepen their understanding of health. As facilitator, you may want to reflect on your own definition of health before teaching this module.

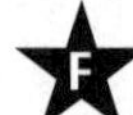

Today's session is the first of two that comprise the Pediatrics in Practice *Health module. This module presents an overview and introduction to the entire* Pediatrics in Practice *curriculum.*

The purpose of this session is to help promote an understanding of health that goes beyond the mere absence of illness or infirmity, and to introduce six concepts that will help you communicate effectively, partner with and educate children and their families, and serve as advocates to promote health and prevent illness in a time-efficient manner.

In today's session, our objectives will be to:
- ▶ *Explore and expand our definition and understanding of the "healthy child"*
- ▶ *Understand the six core concepts addressed in the* Pediatrics in Practice *curriculum*
- ▶ *Gain a greater awareness of how children's health depends on the health of their families and communities*

When we have completed the session, you should be able to answer the following questions:
- ▶ *What is a "healthy" child in the context of the family and community?*
- ▶ *What are the six core concepts that sup-port Bright Futures?*

Discussion and Exercises

The Quick Survey

The facilitator distributes paper to the learners, then reads or paraphrases the following:

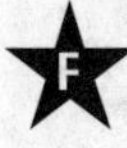 *As child health professionals, you each have definitions of health that determine your expectations about your role in promoting or improving the health of children. Please take 2 or 3 minutes to write down your own definition of a "healthy child."*

While collecting the learners' written responses, the facilitator introduces the Bright Futures videotape and explains, as noted in the introduction, that Bright Futures views health as encompassing not only prevention of morbidity and mortality but also promotion of healthy growth and development, and achievement of the child's full potential.

Bright Futures Videotape— Viewing and Discussion

The facilitator starts the VCR and reviews the learners' survey responses as they watch the videotape. (The run time for the videotape is 16 minutes.)

When the videotape has ended, the facilitator moves to the display board and uses the learners' written responses to engage in a brief discussion on the definition of health. To prompt discussion, the facilitator might ask the following:

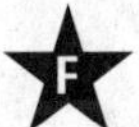 ▶ *In the videotape, how does Bright Futures define health?*

▶ *How are the various definitions similar? How are they different?*

▶ *How does the context of the family's strengths, resources, community, and culture influence your definition of health?*

Overview of Bright Futures and the Core Concepts

The facilitator summarizes the main points of the discussion, relating them to the six core concepts (which the facilitator can briefly describe in any order):

▶ Partnership

▶ Communication

▶ Health Promotion/Illness Prevention

▶ Time Management

▶ Education

▶ Advocacy

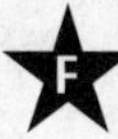 *As described in the videotape, these core concepts are also core competencies or skills that are essential for Bright Futures health professionals to develop in order to help children and their families achieve optimal health.*

Take-Home Message

The facilitator ends the session by summarizing the Bright Futures concept of health:

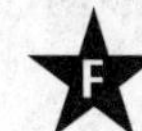 *Health is not only the absence of illness or disease, but also a state of well-being and the opportunity to achieve one's full potential. Bright Futures believes that this can best be achieved by building effective partnerships; fostering family-centered communication; promoting health and preventing illness; managing time for health promotion; educating families through teachable moments; and advocating for children, families, and communities. Before we conclude, what questions remain about what we addressed today?*

Answers to the Guiding Questions

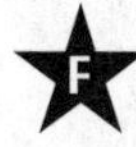 *Now that we have completed this session on Health, you should be able to answer the following questions:*

▶ What is a "healthy" child in the context of the family and community?

• A "healthy" child is able to achieve his or her full potential. The capacity to achieve that potential depends on the strengths and resources of the child, the family, and the community.

▶ What are the six core concepts that support Bright Futures?

• The six core concepts are Partnership, Communication, Health Promotion/Illness Prevention, Time Management, Education, and Advocacy.

Planning for the Next Session (if Session 2 is planned)

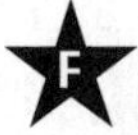 *In the next session, we will explore these core concepts in greater depth, through a case discussion of a well-child visit.*

To prepare for the next session, the facilitator asks the learners to consider the following questions:

▶ How do I, as a pediatric provider, identify the strengths of a child, family, and community?

▶ How do I identify which concerns or agendas should be addressed during the visit?

Evaluation

The facilitator now distributes the **Session Evaluation Form.** The facilitator also completes the **Facilitator Self-Assessment Form.**

Health: Session 1

Bright Futures
Children's Health Charter

Throughout this century, principles developed by advocates for children have been the foundation for initiatives to improve children's lives. Bright Futures participants have adopted these principles in order to guide their work and meet the unique needs of children and families into the 21st century.

Every child deserves to be born well, to be physically fit, and to achieve
self-responsibility for good health habits.

•

Every child and adolescent deserves ready access
to coordinated and comprehensive preventive, health-promoting, therapeutic,
and rehabilitative medical, mental health, and dental care. Such care is best provided
through a continuing relationship with a primary health professional or team,
and ready access to secondary and tertiary levels of care.

•

Every child and adolescent deserves a nurturing family
and supportive relationships with other significant persons who provide security,
positive role models, warmth, love, and unconditional acceptance.
A child's health begins with the health of his parents.

•

Every child and adolescent deserves to grow and develop
in a physically and psychologically safe home and school environment
free of undue risk of injury, abuse, violence, or exposure to environmental toxins.

•

Every child and adolescent deserves satisfactory housing, good nutrition,
a quality education, an adequate family income, a supportive social network,
and access to community resources.

•

Every child deserves quality child care
when her parents are working outside the home.

•

Every child and adolescent deserves the opportunity to develop ways to cope
with stressful life experiences.

•

Every child and adolescent deserves the opportunity to be prepared for parenthood.

•

Every child and adolescent deserves the opportunity to develop positive values
and become a responsible citizen in his community.

•

Every child and adolescent deserves to experience joy, have high self-esteem,
have friends, acquire a sense of efficacy, and believe that she can succeed in life.
She should help the next generation develop the motivation and habits
necessary for similar achievement.

Source: Reproduced with permission from Green M, Palfrey JS, eds. 2002. *Bright Futures: Guidelines for Health Supervision of Infants, Children, and Adolescents* (2nd ed., rev.). Arlington, VA: National Center for Education in Maternal and Child Health.

Health: Session 1

SESSION EVALUATION FORM

Session 1: Health and the Bright Futures Concept

Date: _______________________________

Facilitator(s): _______________________________

Site: _______________________________

---

1. Overall, I found the "Health and the Bright Futures Concept" session to be:

Not Useful				Very Useful
1	2	3	4	5

2. The objectives of the session were:

Not Clear				Clear
1	2	3	4	5

3. The organization of the session was:

Poor				Excellent
1	2	3	4	5

4. The communication skills of the facilitator(s) were:

Poor				Excellent
1	2	3	4	5

5. The facilitator(s) stimulated interest in the subject matter:

Not at All				Very Much
1	2	3	4	5

6. The facilitator(s) encouraged group participation:

Not at All				Very Much
1	2	3	4	5

7. Handouts or visual aids (if used) were:

Not Helpful				Very Helpful
1	2	3	4	5

8. Any additional comments?

____
____
____

9. The most useful features of the session were:

____
____
____

10. Suggestions for improvement

____
____
____

11. Suggestions for topics related to this session

____
____
____

Health: Session 1

FACILITATOR SELF-ASSESSMENT FORM

Directions: Please rate yourself from 1 to 5 on the following facilitator skills. The closer you are to a 5 within each domain, the more skilled you are at facilitation. We encourage you to complete this form prior to and after each teaching experience (e.g., a single session or an entire module). This will allow you to assess your performance as a facilitator over time.

Facilitator Behavior	1	2	3	4	5
Remains neutral					
Does not judge ideas					
Keeps the group focused on common task					
Asks clarifying questions					
Creates a climate free of criticism					
Encourages participation					
Structures participation					

Source: Adapted with permission from Welch, M. (1999). *Teaching diversity and cultural competence in health care: A trainer's guide.* San Francisco, CA: Perspectives of Differences Diversity Training and Consultation for Health Professionals (PODSDT).

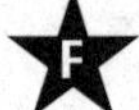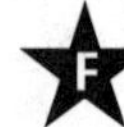

SESSION 2:

Just Another Healthy Child?

At the beginning of the session, the facilitator and learners should introduce themselves briefly. (If the same group has recently completed Session 1, the facilitator may decide that introductions are not needed.) Ideas for creative introductions can be found in the Facilitator's Guide.

Setting the Context: The Bright Futures Concept

(May be omitted if recently presented or when sessions are combined.)

The facilitator **(F)** introduces the learners to the Bright Futures concept of health by reading or paraphrasing the following:

The World Health Organization has defined health as "a state of complete physical, mental and social well-being and not merely the absence of disease or infirmity." Bright Futures embraces this broad definition of health—one that includes not only prevention of morbidity and mortality, but also the achievement of a child's full potential. In the Bright Futures concept of health, providing the capacity for healthy child development is as important as ameliorating illness or injury. Recognizing and acknowledging the strengths and resources of the child, family, and community are essential to promoting healthy growth and development.

To build that capacity, the Pediatrics in Practice *curriculum focuses on six core concepts: Partnership, Communication, Health Promotion/Illness Prevention, Time Management, Education, and Advocacy. The curriculum also includes a companion module (Health) and videotape that present an overview of* Pediatrics in Practice *and the Bright Futures approach.*

Introducing the Session

Today's session is the second of two that comprise the Pediatrics in Practice *Health module. In the last session, we introduced six core concepts: Partnership, Communication, Health Promotion/Illness Prevention, Time Manage-ment, Education, and Advocacy. This session illustrates these concepts in greater depth and provides opportunities to build or practice related skills.*

In today's session, our objectives will be to:

▶ *Gain a better understanding of the importance of acknowledging the strengths of the child, family, and community as partners in health*

▶ *Identify the child's, family's, and health professional's concerns or agendas during a health visit*

▶ *Recognize the health professional's role in supporting families and communities in promoting children's health*

When we have completed this session, you should be able to answer the following questions:

▶ *How do I, as a pediatric provider, identify the strengths of a child, family, and community?*

▶ *How do I identify which concerns or agendas should be addressed during a health visit?*

Discussion and Exercises

The facilitator distributes copies of the handout **Case Vignette: Janice's 10 Year Visit**, as well as the handouts **Bright Futures Interview Questions for 10 Year Visit** and **Case Growth Chart**. The facilitator asks one of the learners to read the case vignette handout aloud.

Case Discussion

The facilitator moves to the display board and opens the discussion as follows:

This case represents a "normal" or typical well-child visit; however, as we will see, the child health professional can do a lot to help the child continue healthy habits and achieve healthy development during the approaching adolescent years. In addition to the case vignette, I've provided two other handouts (interview questions and growth chart) as examples of resources that can serve as effective health promotion tools. The health interview is drawn from the Bright Futures interview questions for the 10 year visit, and helps elicit many issues that the health professional needs to be aware of. The CDC growth chart can be both a clinical and educational tool, as the health professional plots the child's height and weight on the chart, shares the information with the family, and uses this "teachable moment" to reinforce the importance of healthy eating and physical activity in achieving optimal growth and development. The growth chart also demonstrates the importance of continuity of care, since data from previous visits are needed to properly assess the child's growth and development.

As child health professionals, we usually consider ourselves "trouble shooters" and problem-solvers, but we also need to recognize and acknowledge the strengths of children and their families. This exercise is meant to build the family's confidence in their capacity to resolve their own issues and problems.

Based on the information in the handout, what strengths can you identify in the case of Janice and her family?

The facilitator waits at least 1 minute for learners to answer, then writes their responses on the display board. If necessary, the facilitator prompts the discussion by mentioning a few items from the list below:

Janice's strengths
▶ Has intact and supportive family
▶ Feels safe
▶ Achieves good academic performance in school
▶ Has a positive disposition
▶ Likes to read

▶ Enjoys physical activity (bike riding)
▶ Has plans for the future
▶ Interacts well with peers

After identifying these (and possibly other) strengths, the facilitator explains that each person in the exam room has an agenda for the visit. Sometimes, in an effort to complete the health promotion goals or agenda for the visit, the child health professional may not address all of the family's concerns. Or the child's agenda may be ignored because he or she is not given ample opportunity to speak. Recognizing each person's agenda for the visit can improve communication and promote partnership between the professional, the child, and the family.

After explaining the importance of recognizing each person's agenda, the facilitator then asks the learners:

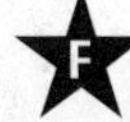

Again, based on the handout, can you identify the three agendas for the health visit—Janice's, her father's, and your own?

Using the display board, the facilitator sets up three columns with headings, as below. If necessary, the facilitator can prompt discussion by citing some possible responses:

Extended Discussion and Exercises (optional)

If time permits, the facilitator can guide in-depth discussion on key issues presented in the case vignette, such as prioritizing health agendas, approaching adolescence, or providing a safe after-school environment.

Prioritizing Agendas

The facilitator can pose this question to the learners and note their responses:

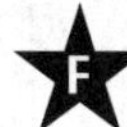

How do you plan to address these differing agendas during this health visit? How will you use your knowledge of the child's and family's strengths to address these issues?

After listing some of the learners' responses on the display board, the facilitator might emphasize that the Bright Futures guidelines can sometimes appear overwhelming because they address such a broad range of health promotion and illness prevention issues. Even a typical

JANICE	FATHER	HEALTH PROFESSIONAL
• Getting a shot?	• Shots up to date?	• Immunizations
• Neighbor's pipe	• Child care and home safety	• Child care
• Mean kid	• Health care coverage	• Anti-smoking counseling
• Fat?	• Ways to discuss puberty	• Encouraging reading
	• Janice healthy?	• Safety promotion
		• Adolescence and body image
		• Healthy eating habits
		• Physical activity
		• Peer relations
		• Completing chart
		• Staying on schedule

well-child visit such as the one described in the case vignette provides opportunities to address more issues than time may allow. The key is to elicit the agendas of the child, family, and health professional, then set priorities for this visit and perhaps follow-up visits based on the three agendas.

Approaching Adolescence

The facilitator might also ask the learners:

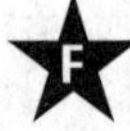 *How would you answer the question raised by Janice's father concerning her "growing up"? (That is, how would you help him address or anticipate adolescence issues?)*

Learners can explore how they would help Janice's parents talk with her about adolescence issues such as sexuality and substance use. The facilitator may also want to point out parent and patient education materials available at the learners' clinic sites. One core component of Bright Futures health supervision is anticipatory guidance, which helps families plan for the future growth and development of their child.

Providing a Safe After-School Environment

Addressing another topic that can be drawn from the case, the facilitator might state:

 *Janice's father was concerned about the lack of affordable child care for his children. How could you as a child health professional help address this problem?*

This question may generate a range of responses, and the facilitator should explain that the absence of quality child care is a problem that typically cannot be adequately handled in the health professional's office or clinic. Bright Futures recognizes that the health of the child also depends on the health of families and communities, and that the child health professional has a role beyond that of caring for children in a practice. Learners might discuss their role as pediatric providers in promoting health in children, and talk about how they can become effective child advocates. For example, the health professional could advocate for after-school programs through the school or through community organizations.

What Is a "Healthy Child"?

In concluding discussion on this topic, the facilitator might return to the original topic in Session 1 by asking:

 *Is Janice healthy? How can you as child health professionals help Janice optimize her health?*

Session 1 examined Bright Futures concepts and the definition of "healthy." Using the learners' own definitions, the facilitator asks them to consider whether Janice is "healthy." Based on the Bright Futures concept of health, the facilitator can challenge learners to discuss other strategies and action steps they could use to promote Janice's health.

Take-Home Message

The facilitator ends the session with the following:

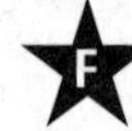 *Even a "normal" well-child visit presents frequent opportunities to increase the capacity of the child and family to improve their health. Acknowledging the child's and family's strengths and identifying their agendas is the first step toward becoming an effective Bright Futures health professional. Before we conclude, what questions remain about what we addressed today?*

Answers to the Guiding Questions

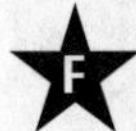 *Now that we have completed this session on Health, you should be able to answer the following questions:*

▶ How do I, as a pediatric provider, identify the strengths of a child, family, and community?

  - Identifying strengths means recognizing the capacity of the child, family, and community to address challenges. Strengths can include values, knowledge, skills, or resources. All of these can be used to promote the health and development of the child.

▶ How do I identify which concerns or agendas should be addressed during a health visit?

  - First, recognize the differing agendas of the child, parents, and health professional, as illustrated in discussion of the case vignette. Then, prioritize these agendas and address the child's and parent's top priority needs. This will ensure good communication and build an effective partnership with the family.

Evaluation

The facilitator now distributes the **Session Evaluation Form.** The facilitator also completes the **Facilitator Self-Assessment Form.**

Health: Session 2

CASE VIGNETTE:
JANICE'S 10 YEAR VISIT

Janice, accompanied by her father, has come for her scheduled 10 year well-child visit. Scanning her record, you note that Janice has had regular health supervision visits throughout infancy and childhood, with a few visits for viral illnesses. Her immunizations are up to date, and her previous screening tests are all in the normal range.

Janice and her father give you a cheery hello as you enter the exam room and ask Janice, "How are you today?"

"I'm fine," Janice replies. She tells you that she is in now in the fifth grade and likes school. She lives with her parents, her 7-year-old brother, Juan, and their dog. No one at home smokes, but a neighbor smokes a pipe, which smells "yucky." Janice then asks, "Am I going to get a shot today?"

Janice's father says, "Janice is pretty healthy, but I want to be sure she has had all of her shots."

You explain to Janice and her father that she has had all of the recommended childhood immunizations so she doesn't need any "catch-up" vaccinations, but that in the next year or two she'll need another shot for tetanus and then routine "boosters" every 10 years, just like adults.

You recall that Janice's father works as a legal assistant at a law firm, and that her mother works as a receptionist at a dentist's office. Since neither employer offers health insurance for dependents, Janice and her brother receive health care coverage through the State Children's Health Insurance Program (SCHIP). Janice's father is concerned that Janice and her brother are alone for about an hour after school every day until one of the parents arrives home, but they can't afford child care expenses. The parents have taught the children home safety rules, and they try to limit television viewing to 1 hour on weekdays.

Janice likes to ride her bicycle with her best friend, Caren, and to read stories on the weekends. She has lots of other friends at school. She wants to be a lawyer or president of the United States when she grows up. She feels safe at home and school, although she mentions a boy at school who is "mean" and calls her "fatso."

During her physical exam, Janice appears healthy and enthusiastic. Both her hearing and vision are in the normal range, and the examination yields no abnormal findings. Her height is at the 50th percentile and her weight at the 75th percentile for her age. Developmentally, Janice's sexual maturity rating is assessed at Tanner stage 2.

After the physical exam has been completed, Janice's father asks, "When should her mother and I talk to Janice about growing up? I'm not sure what to say."

Health: Session 2

BRIGHT FUTURES INTERVIEW QUESTIONS FOR 10 YEAR VISIT

Questions for the Parent(s)

- How does Sanjay express his feelings and share his experiences with you?
- What are some of the things you do together as a family?
- How much time does he spend watching TV? On the computer?
- What is his bedtime?
- What have you discussed with Nancy about her changing body?
- What has she learned about menstruation?

Questions for the Child

- How is school going? How are your grades?
- Tell me about your friends. What do you like to do together? What activities are you involved in?
- Do your friends pressure you to do things you don't want to do? What kinds of things?
- How do you get along with your family? With your teachers?
- What education have you had about sex? What are some of the questions I can answer for you?
- What do you like to eat? Are you concerned about your weight? Are you trying to change it?
- What are some things that make you happy? Sad? Angry? Worried? Who do you talk to about them?

Development and School Performance

- What changes have you noticed in Pablo's behavior, relationships, or school performance? Do you have concerns about his development or behavior?
- Has he identified certain interests or talents he would like to develop?
- Is Pablo reading and doing math at grade level?
- Tell me about his grades.
- Where and how does Pablo do his homework?

Observation: Do both parent and child ask questions? Does parent interrupt when child is speaking to health professional? Is child comfortable if health professional speaks with him alone?

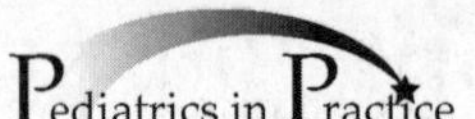

Health: Session 2

CASE GROWTH CHART

Two to 20 years: Girls
Stature-for-age and Weight-for-age percentiles

NAME ____________________

RECORD __________

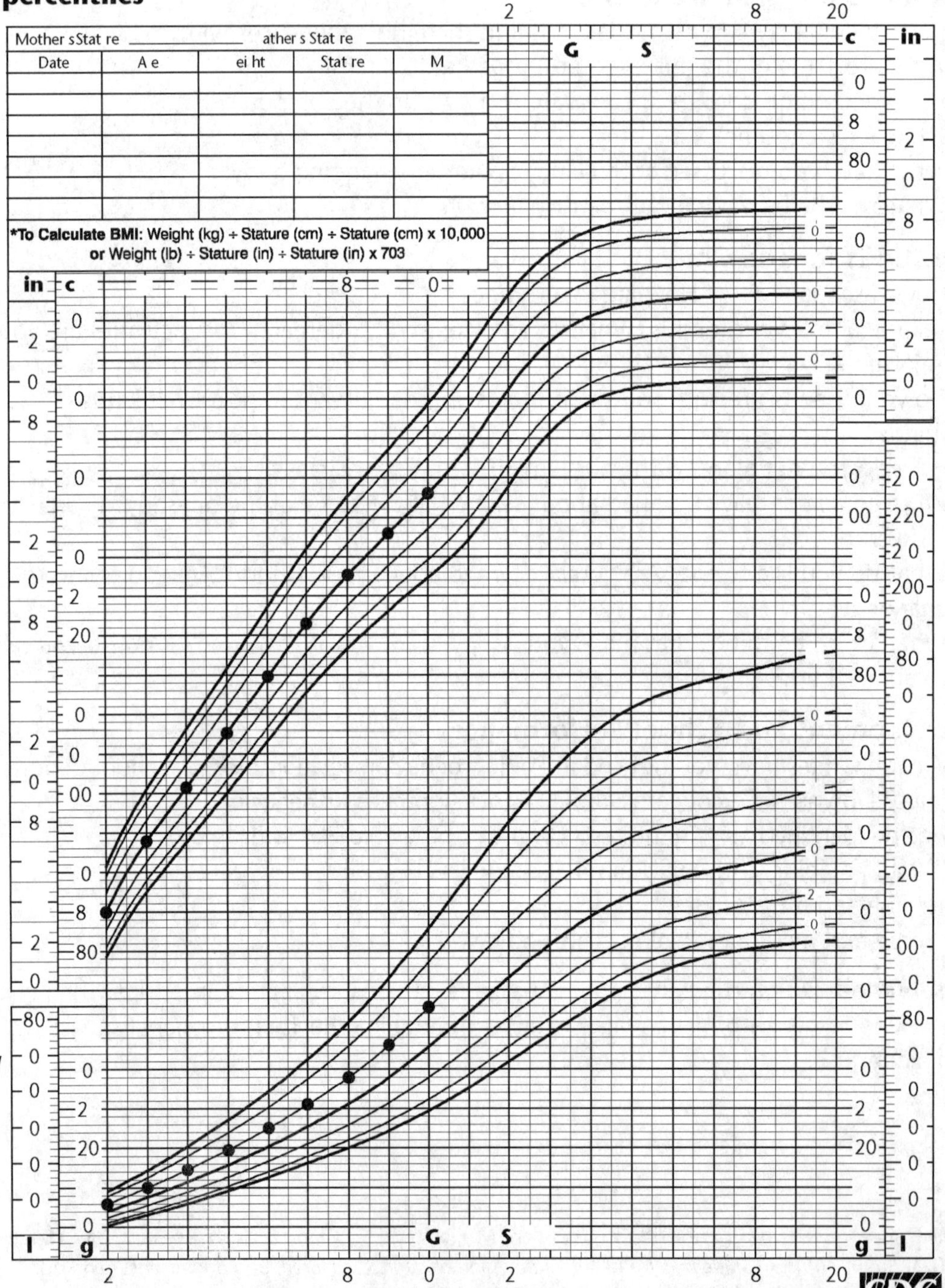

Source: Developed by the National Center for Health Statistics in collaboration with the National Center for Chronic Disease Prevention and Health Promotion (2000). **http://www.cdc.gov/growthcharts**
Revised and Corrected November 28, 2000.

Health: Session 2

SESSION EVALUATION FORM

Session 2: Just Another Healthy Child?

Date: ________________________

Facilitator(s): ________________________

Site: ________________________

---

1. Overall, I found the "Just Another Healthy Child?" session to be:	**Not Useful** **Very Useful** 1 2 3 4 5	
2. The objectives of the session were:	**Not Clear** **Clear** 1 2 3 4 5	
3. The organization of the session was:	**Poor** **Excellent** 1 2 3 4 5	
4. The communication skills of the facilitator(s) were:	**Poor** **Excellent** 1 2 3 4 5	
5. The facilitator(s) stimulated interest in the subject matter:	**Not at All** **Very Much** 1 2 3 4 5	
6. The facilitator(s) encouraged group participation:	**Not at All** **Very Much** 1 2 3 4 5	
7. Handouts or visual aids (if used) were:	**Not Helpful** **Very Helpful** 1 2 3 4 5	

8. Any additional comments?

____

____

____

9. The most useful features of the session were:

____

____

____

10. Suggestions for improvement

____

____

____

11. Suggestions for topics related to this session

____

____

____

Health: Session 2

FACILITATOR SELF-ASSESSMENT FORM

Directions: Please rate yourself from 1 to 5 on the following facilitator skills. The closer you are to a 5 within each domain, the more skilled you are at facilitation. We encourage you to complete this form prior to and after each teaching experience (e.g., a single session or an entire module). This will allow you to assess your performance as a facilitator over time.

Facilitator Behavior	1	2	3	4	5
Remains neutral					
Does not judge ideas					
Keeps the group focused on common task					
Asks clarifying questions					
Creates a climate free of criticism					
Encourages participation					
Structures participation					

Source: Adapted with permission from Welch, M. (1999). *Teaching diversity and cultural competence in health care: A trainer's guide.* San Francisco, CA: Perspectives of Differences Diversity Training and Consultation for Health Professionals (PODSDT).

References

American Academy of Pediatrics (1992). The medical home. *Pediatrics, 90,* 774.

American Academy of Pediatrics, Committee on Community Health Services (1999). The pediatrician's role in community pediatrics. *Pediatrics, 103,* 1304–1306.

American Academy of Pediatrics, Committee on Psychosocial Aspects of Child and Family Health (1993). The pediatrician and the "new morbidity." *Pediatrics, 92,* 731–733.

Benjamin, J.T., Cimino, S.A., & Hafler, J.P., Bright Futures Health Promotion Work Group, Bernstein, H.H. (2002). The office visit: A time to promote health—but how? *Contemporary Pediatrics, 19*(2), 90–107.

Bonfield, A. (prod.) (2000). *Bright futures: Health supervision of infants, children, and adolescents* [videotape, part of the *Pediatrics in Practice* health promotion curriculum]. Sharon, MA: Biomedical Video and Multimedia.

Centers for Disease Control and Prevention (2000). *2000 CDC growth charts: United States.* [Developed by the National Center for Health Statistics in collaboration with the National Center for Chronic Disease Prevention and Health Promotion.] Available online at www.cdc.gov/growthcharts.

Green, M., & Palfrey, J.S. (Eds.) (2002). *Bright futures: Guidelines for health supervision of infants, children, and adolescents* (2nd ed., rev.). Arlington, VA: National Center for Education in Maternal and Child Health.

Green, M., Palfrey, J.S., Clark, E.M., & Anastasi, J.M. (Eds.) (2002). *Bright futures: Guidelines for health supervision of infants, children, and adolescents* (2nd ed., rev.)—*Pocket guide.* Arlington, VA: National Center for Education in Maternal and Child Health.

Palfrey, J.S. (1994). *Community child health: An action plan for today.* Westport, CT: Praeger Publishers.

World Health Organization (1978). *Primary health care.* Report of the International Conference on Primary Health Care, Alma Ata, USSR. Geneva: World Health Organization.

Resources

Ambulatory Pediatrics Association Web site: www.ambpeds.org.

American Academy of Pediatrics. (1994). *TIPP: The injury prevention program.* Elk Grove Village, IL: American Academy of Pediatrics.

American Academy of Pediatrics, Committee on Practice and Ambulatory Medicine. 2000. Recommendations for preventive pediatric health care. *Pediatrics, 105*(3), 645.

American Academy of Pediatrics, Committee on Psychosocial Aspects of Child and Family Health. (2002). *Guidelines for health supervision III.* Elk Grove Village, IL: American Academy of Pediatrics.

American Academy of Pediatrics Web site: www.aap.org.

Bright Futures Web site: www.brightfutures.org.

Family Voices Web site: www.familyvoices.org.

Zero to Three Web site: www.zerotothree.org.

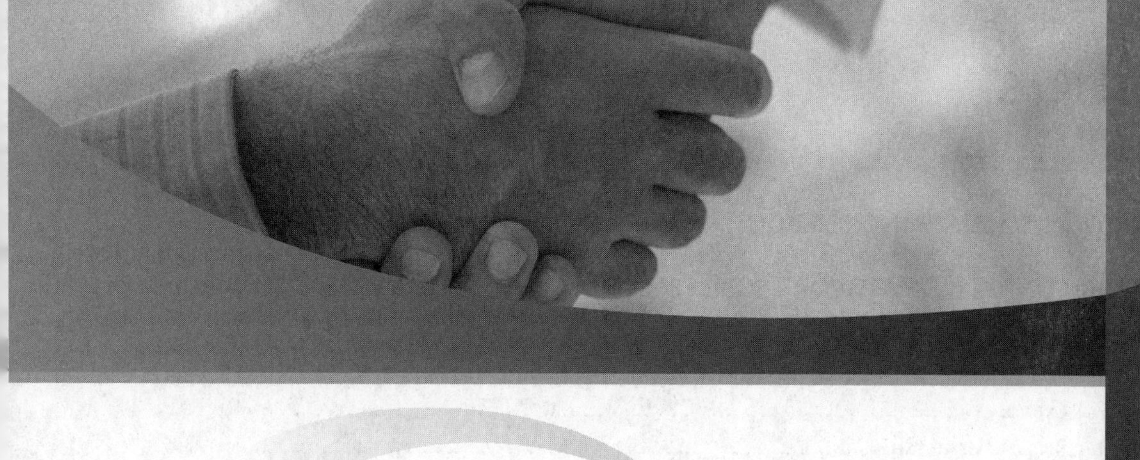

Partnership

Building Effective Partnerships

Danielle Laraque

Joe Lopreiato

Diane Pickles

CONTENTS

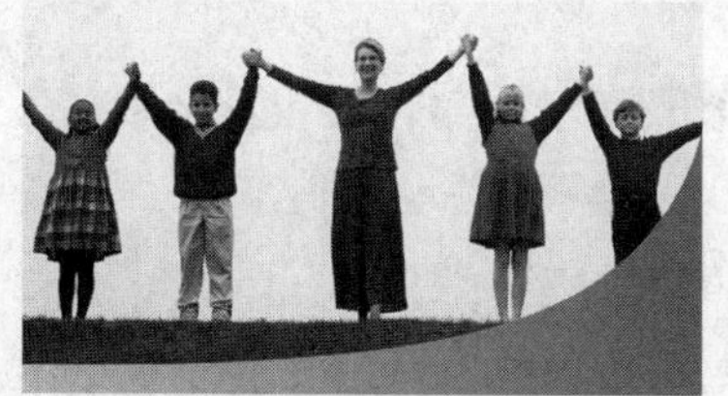

PARTNERSHIP
Building Effective Partnerships

OVERVIEW

Background

Many child health professionals are not used to assessing family and community strengths during health visits and may be unfamiliar with the concept of partnering with the family and/or community to address health issues. Building an effective partnership with a family or community can be a powerful tool in promoting health, reducing disparities in care, and developing realistic treatment goals. In the context of health maintenance, partnership-building promotes child wellness and is an essential ingredient for family satisfaction with care.

Goal

The overall goals of this module are to increase child health professionals' awareness of the importance and benefits of partnering with families and communities, and to enable professionals to develop the knowledge, attitudes, and skills necessary to build and sustain partnerships.

This module will enable learners to:

▶ Understand the six essential steps in developing collaborative, productive partnerships with families and communities

▶ Increase their awareness of the attitudes or qualities needed to develop effective partnerships

▶ Build the skills necessary for developing successful partnerships among health professionals, children, and families

Instructional Design

This module consists of two 30-minute sessions.

▶ Session 1 identifies important attitudes and qualities that enhance partnerships, and introduces the six essential steps in partnership building.

▶ Session 2 offers an in-depth look at developing partnership skills, using the six-step framework.

▶ Each of the two sessions can be used as a separate stand-alone offering, or the sessions can be combined. See the Facilitator's Guide for information on combining sessions.

Teaching Strategies

The teaching strategies used in this module include case discussion, reflective exercise, and brainstorming. These strategies have been selected to help learners develop the skills required to build effective partnerships between child health professionals and families. Please refer to the Facilitator's Guide for more information related to each strategy.

Evaluation

Learners will complete a **Session Evaluation Form** following each session. Facilitators are encouraged to complete a **Facilitator Self-Assessment Form** prior to and following each teaching experience (e.g., a single session or an entire module) in order to assess their performance over time.

Guiding Questions

Learners who have completed the entire Partnership module should be able to answer the following questions:

▶ What specific attitudes do child health professionals need in order to adopt the Bright Futures philosophy and to effectively partner with families?

- What are some of the major benefits of building an effective partnership with a child and family?
- What are the six essential steps for building effective partnerships?
- How do open-ended and culturally sensitive interview questions facilitate communication between the child health professional and the family?
- How can child health professionals work in partnership with families to promote health, identify problems, and implement solutions?
- What specific skills do child health professionals need in order to foster more effective partnerships with children, families, and/or communities?
- Of the six steps for building partnerships, which step is most critical in building a partnership with the family?

INTRODUCTION TO TEACHING SESSIONS

Session 1: Building a Framework for Effective Partnerships

Objectives

The objectives for this session are for the facilitator to:

- Help learners gain a greater awareness of the attitudes or qualities needed to form partnerships with families and communities
- Introduce the six-step model for building effective health partnerships

Materials

The materials and teaching aids needed for this session are:

Handouts
- Partnership: Building Effective Partnerships
- Session Evaluation Form

Facilitator Form
- Facilitator Self-Assessment Form

Teaching Aids
- Display board, flip chart, or chalkboard
- Markers or chalk
- Blank 3" x 5" index cards

Time

The time allocated for this session is 30 minutes.

Session 2: Skills Training: Applying the Six Steps of Partnership

Objectives

The objectives for this session are for the facilitator to:
- Guide learners through a practical application of the six essential steps in partnership
- Help learners build the skills needed to develop successful partnerships between child health professionals, children, and families

Materials

The materials and teaching aids needed for this session are:

Handouts
- Partnership: Building Effective Partnerships
- Case Vignette: The Montes Family
- Case Discussion: Applying the Six Steps of Partnership
- On Listening
- Session Evaluation Form

Facilitator Form
- Facilitator Self-Assessment Form

Teaching Aids
- Display board, flip chart, or chalkboard
- Markers or chalk

Time

The time allocated for this session is 30 minutes.

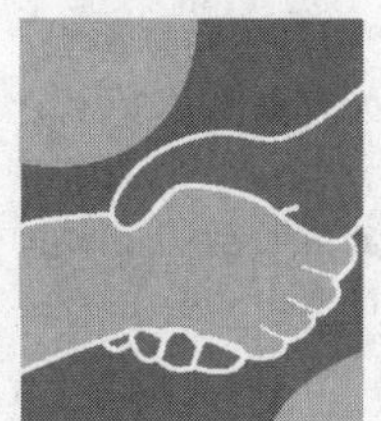

SESSION 1:
Building a Framework for Effective Partnerships

At the beginning of the session, the facilitator and learners should introduce themselves briefly. Ideas for creative introductions can be found in the Facilitator's Guide.

Setting the Context: The Bright Futures Concept

The facilitator **(F)** introduces the learners to the Bright Futures concept of health by reading or paraphrasing the following:

The World Health Organization has defined health as "a state of complete physical, mental and social well-being and not merely the absence of disease or infirmity." Bright Futures embraces this broad definition of health—one that includes not only prevention of morbidity and mortality, but also the achievement of a child's full potential. In the Bright Futures concept of health, providing the capacity for healthy child development is as important as ameliorating illness or injury. Recognizing and acknowledging the strengths and resources of the child, family, and community are essential to promoting healthy growth and development.

To build that capacity, the Pediatrics in Practice *curriculum focuses on six core concepts: Partnership, Communication, Health Promotion/Illness Prevention, Time Management, Education, and Advocacy. The curriculum also includes a companion module (Health) and videotape that present an overview of* Pediatrics in Practice *and the Bright Futures approach.*

Introducing the Session

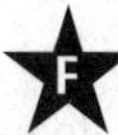

Today's session is the first of two that comprise the Partnership module. For some of you, the concept of a clinical partnership is relatively new; for others, the concept is familiar, but a method for developing partnerships in your practice may be new.

The principles of partnering can be applied at the individual or community level. This module focuses on fostering individual partnerships between child health professionals and the children and families they serve. However, similar concepts may be applied to community partnerships. (The Advocacy module explores important concepts in partnering with communities.)

Today's module introduces a conceptual framework for clinical partnerships: six steps that help build and maintain successful partnerships in your practice.

In today's session, our objectives will be to:

▶ *Explore key attitudes or qualities that are prerequisites for building effective partnerships*

▶ *Introduce a six-step framework for developing clinical partnerships*

When we have completed the session, you should be able to answer the following questions:

▶ *What specific attitudes do child health professionals need in order to adopt the Bright Futures approach?*

▶ *What are some of the major benefits of building a successful partnership with a child and family?*

▶ *What are the six essential steps for building effective partnerships?*

Discussion and Exercises

Defining a Clinical Partnership

The facilitator may choose to write the following definition on the display board while presenting it to the learners:

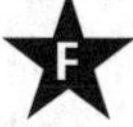

For working purposes, let us define a clinical partnership as the delivery of health care in a

Reflective Exercise, Part 1: Aspects and Attributes of Partnerships

The facilitator hands out 3" x 5" cards to the learners and asks them to list the characteristics or attributes that create a successful partnership between the health professional, the child, and the family. Learners are encouraged to draw from their own health care encounters, if possible, to list provider and/or family attributes that have made a clinical relationship especially effective.

Specifically, the facilitator asks the following questions to prompt discussion:

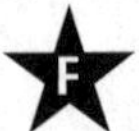

▶ *What characteristics of the child health professional might facilitate a clinical partnership?*

▶ *What patient or family characteristics might help foster the partnership?*

The facilitator then asks each learner to offer one characteristic of a successful partnership, from the health professional's or the family's perspective.

The facilitator lists responses on the display board. Possible responses include the following:

Reflective Exercise, Part 2: Barriers and Benefits to Partnering

The facilitator acknowledges some specific barriers to partnering by reading or paraphrasing the following:

Developing partnerships begins with attitudes, but sometimes attitudes present potential barriers. Some families, for example, are reluctant to partner and prefer to follow the health professional's recommendations. Sometimes, either the health professional or the family believes that an equal partnership is not possible because professionals have the medical knowledge that families lack; others may think the health visit is more "efficient" when the professional decides on a plan of action and clearly explains it to the family. Time constraints, too, can be persuasive in convincing some health professionals that attempting to partner with every family is unrealistic and takes too much time.

The facilitator then explains that barriers to partnership can be reexamined in the context of potential benefits, and asks the learners to list some major benefits of partnering, again drawing on their clinical experience but also on their observations or suggestions. Possible responses include the following:

▶ Parents have a lot to contribute to the care and well-being of their child.

▶ The child health professional may overlook an important health or developmental concern unless the family is involved in care.

▶ Home health management is easier when the family helps decide on the plan of action.

▶ Adherence to a health care plan is most likely when the family is actively involved.

▶ Health professionals can avoid making assumptions or generalizations that may not apply to a particular family, and are better able to target health promotion to the

From the Child Health Professional	From the Child and Parent
• Be open	• Have a strong interest in the child's health and well-being
• Be willing to listen	
• Have a nonjudgmental attitude	• Demonstrate interest in one's own health (adolescent)
• Be knowledgeable	
• Be respectful	• Trust the relationship with the health professional
• Demonstrate genuine interest in and understanding of the child and family	
	• Be on time
• Engender trust	• Be prepared
• Express empathy	• Ask thoughtful questions
• Display willingness to negotiate and understand other perspectives	• Try to understand aspects of health in detail
• Be on time	• Be able to disagree with a proposed health plan and suggest alternative strategies
• Ask questions that invite more than a yes/no answer	

unique needs of the family, when a partnership is formed.

The Six Essential Steps in Partnering

The facilitator distributes the handout **Partnership: Building Effective Partnerships** and states:

 *As we conclude this session, I want to move beyond key attitudes and introduce a practical set of steps that form the framework for building partnerships with children and their families. In the next session, we will develop some skill-building tools to put these steps into practice in the health visit.*

Take-Home Message

The facilitator summarizes by reading or paraphrasing:

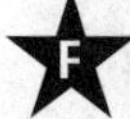 *Partnership development is a continuum, from sharing information to partnering around certain issues to building a full partnership in health. The key to building a partnership is to recognize that all children and families possess information and skills critical to optimal health care delivery.*

Families who partner with their health professional participate more fully in health care delivery. They feel more comfortable sharing information with the professional and are more committed to following through with an identified health care plan.

Creating or sustaining full partnerships with individual patients and families is not always easy or even possible. Family dynamics, personalities, and other issues may prevent providers and families from participating as equal partners. However, it is important to consistently nurture the elements of trust, respect, and empathy in every relationship. These qualities—some of which will be addressed in Session 2 of this module—ultimately foster an effective partnership. They help prevent the frustration and conflict that can ultimately lead to poor time management and ineffective health care delivery. Before we conclude, what questions remain about what we addressed today?

Answers to the Guiding Questions

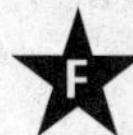 *Now that we have competed this session on Partnership, you should be able to answer the following questions:*

▶ What specific attitudes do child health professionals need in order to adopt the Bright Futures approach?

- Health professionals need to develop attitudes that foster trusting, empathic, respectful relationships between the professional and the children and families they serve. Openness, a willingness to actively listen, and the capacity to learn from and affirm the child's and family's strengths are critical.

▶ What are some of the major benefits of building a successful partnership with a child and family?

- Improved quality of care for the child is one of the best outcomes of forming true partnerships with families. This quality of care is reflected in prompt and accurate identification of family concerns, appropriate management and follow-up of identified problems, efficient use of the family's and the professional's time, and family satisfaction with care.

▶ What are the six essential steps for building effective partnerships?

- Model and encourage open, supportive communication with the child and family.
- Identify issues through active listening and "fact finding."
- Affirm the strengths of the child and family.
- Identify shared goals.
- Develop a joint plan of action based on stated goals.
- Follow up: Sustain the partnership.

Planning for the Next Session (if Session 2 is planned)

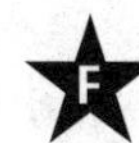 *In the next session, we will use the six-step framework in a case discussion in order to develop practical skills in building partnerships in the health encounter.*

To prepare for the next session, the facilitator asks the learners to consider the following questions:

▶ How do open-ended and culturally sensitive interview questions facilitate communication between the child health professional and the family?

▶ How can child health professionals work in partnership with families to promote health, identify problems, and implement solutions?

▶ What specific skills do child health professionals need in order to foster more effective partnerships with children, families, and/or communities?

▶ Of the six steps for building partnerships, which step is most critical in building a partnership with the family?

Evaluation

The facilitator now distributes the **Session Evaluation Form.** The facilitator also completes the **Facilitator Self-Assessment Form.**

Partnership: Session 1

PARTNERSHIP: BUILDING EFFECTIVE PARTNERSHIPS

A clinical partnership is a relationship in which participants join together to ensure health care delivery in a way that recognizes the critical roles and contributions of each partner (child, family, health professional, and community) in promoting health and preventing illness. Following are six steps for building effective health partnerships.

1. Model and encourage open, supportive communication with child and family.
- Integrate family-centered communication strategies
- Use communication skills to build trust, respect, and empathy

2. Identify health issues through active listening and "fact finding."
- Selectively choose Bright Futures general and age-appropriate interview questions
- Ask open-ended questions to encourage more complete sharing of information
- Communicate understanding of the issues and provide feedback

3. Affirm strengths of child and family.
- Recognize what each person brings to the partnership
- Acknowledge and respect each person's contributions
- Commend family for specific health and developmental achievements

4. Identify shared goals.
- Promote view of health supervision as partnership between child, family, health professional, and community
- Summarize mutual goals
- Provide links between stated goals, health issues, and available resources in community

5. Develop joint plan of action based on stated goals.
- Be sure that each partner has a role in developing the plan
- Keep plan simple and achievable
- Set measurable goals and specific timeline
- Use family-friendly negotiation skills to ensure agreement
- Build in mechanism and time for follow-up

6. Follow up: Sustaining the partnership.
- Share progress, successes, and challenges
- Evaluate and adjust plan
- Provide ongoing support and resources

Partnership: Session 1

SESSION EVALUATION FORM

Session 1: Building a Framework for Effective Partnerships

Date: _________________________________

Facilitator(s): ____

Site: ____

---

1. Overall, I found the "Building a Framework for Effective Partnerships" session to be:

Not Useful			Very Useful	
1	2	3	4	5

2. The objectives of the session were:

Not Clear				Clear
1	2	3	4	5

3. The organization of the session was:

Poor				Excellent
1	2	3	4	5

4. The communication skills of the facilitator(s) were:

Poor				Excellent
1	2	3	4	5

5. The facilitator(s) stimulated interest in the subject matter:

Not at All			Very Much	
1	2	3	4	5

6. The facilitator(s) encouraged group participation:

Not at All			Very Much	
1	2	3	4	5

7. Handouts or visual aids (if used) were:

Not Helpful		Very Helpful		
1	2	3	4	5

8. Any additional comments?

____
____
____

9. The most useful features of the session were:

____
____
____

10. Suggestions for improvement

____
____
____

11. Suggestions for topics related to this session

____
____
____

Partnership: Session 1

FACILITATOR SELF-ASSESSMENT FORM

Directions: Please rate yourself from 1 to 5 on the following facilitator skills. The closer you are to a 5 within each domain, the more skilled you are at facilitation. We encourage you to complete this form prior to and after each teaching experience (e.g., a single session or an entire module). This will allow you to assess your performance as a facilitator over time.

Facilitator Behavior	1	2	3	4	5
Remains neutral					
Does not judge ideas					
Keeps the group focused on common task					
Asks clarifying questions					
Creates a climate free of criticism					
Encourages participation					
Structures participation					

Source: Adapted with permission from Welch, M. (1999). *Teaching diversity and cultural competence in health care: A trainer's guide.* San Francisco, CA: Perspectives of Differences Diversity Training and Consultation for Health Professionals (PODSDT).

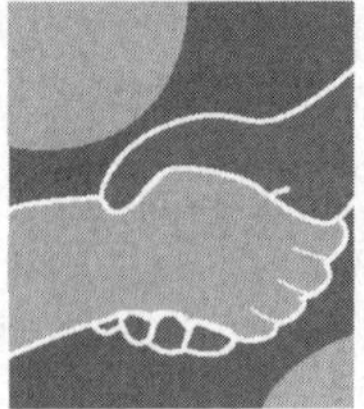

SESSION 2:

Skills Training: Applying the Six Steps of Partnerships

At the beginning of the session, the facilitator and learners should introduce themselves briefly. (If the same group has recently completed Session 1, the facilitator may decide that introductions are not needed.) Ideas for creative introductions can be found in the Facilitator's Guide.

Setting the Context: The Bright Futures Concept

(May be omitted if recently presented or when sessions are combined.)

The facilitator **(F)** introduces the learners to the Bright Futures concept of health by reading or paraphrasing the following:

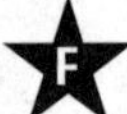 *The World Health Organization has defined health as "a state of complete physical, mental and social well-being and not merely the absence of disease or infirmity." Bright Futures embraces this broad definition of health—one that includes not only prevention of morbidity and mortality, but also the achievement of a child's full potential. In the Bright Futures concept of health, providing the capacity for healthy child development is as important as ameliorating illness or injury. Recognizing and acknowledging the strengths and resources of the child, family, and community are essential to promoting healthy growth and development.*

To build that capacity, the Pediatrics in Practice *curriculum focuses on six core concepts: Partnership, Communication, Health Promotion/Illness Prevention, Time Management, Education, and Advocacy. The curriculum also includes a companion module (Health) and videotape that present an overview of* Pediatrics in Practice *and the Bright Futures approach.*

Introducing the Session

 *During the first session, we examined the core attitudes and six essential steps that support the development of clinical partnerships. This session is designed to help you build the skills needed to develop successful partnerships. We will focus on building those skills through practical application of the six steps in the context of the health visit.*

In this session, our objectives will be to:

▶ *Review the six essential steps for building clinical partnerships*

▶ *Practice the skills needed to develop effective partnerships between child health professionals, children, and families*

When we have completed the session, you should be able to answer the following questions:

▶ *How do open-ended and culturally sensitive interview questions facilitate communication between the child health professional and the family?*

▶ *How can child health professionals work in partnership with families to promote health, identify problems, and implement solutions?*

▶ *What specific skills do child health professionals need in order to foster more effective partnerships with children, families, and/or communities?*

▶ *Of the six steps for building partnerships, which step is most critical in building a partnership with the family?*

Discussion and Exercises

The facilitator distributes the handout **Partnership: Building Effective Partnerships.**

 *In the last session, we introduced the six essential steps to effective partnering. This session "fleshes out" those steps and pres-*

ents practical ways to apply them in a health encounter.

The facilitator reads or paraphrases the following:

Partnering is an ongoing process—health professionals cannot work their way through the steps once and expect the process to be complete. Building and sustaining effective partnerships means continuing to "work the steps on an ongoing basis."

Skills in time management and prioritizing goals (covered in the Time Management module) are also critical in being able to complete the six steps of partnership. Once the building blocks of partnership are in place, a successful partnership can enhance the time available for health promotion.

Let's look at specific partnership skills through a case vignette.

Case Vignette: The Montes Family

The facilitator distributes the handout **Case Vignette: The Montes Family**, then asks one of the learners to read the case aloud.

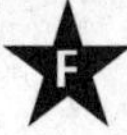

Developing a clinical partnership is not a simple skill. Asking open-ended questions, carefully listening to the family to elicit their concerns, communicating in an understanding and supportive way, recognizing and affirming the family's strengths and unique contributions, establishing mutual goals, and developing an action plan—all involve complex skills that require practice.

In this segment, we will use a case vignette to provide practice in building those partnership skills.

Case Discussion

The facilitator distributes the handout **Case Discussion: Applying the Six Steps of Partnership**, then guides the learners through a step-by-step application of the partnership model.

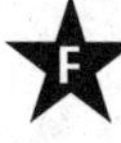

Using the case vignette and the follow-up questions I've just handed out, let's "work the steps" to begin developing a partnership with Ms. Montes and Moses.

With the discussion questions in mind, let's

consider the Montes case through the six-step framework for building partnerships.

Step 1: Model and Encourage Open, Supportive Communication with the Child and Family

Note that we want to emphasize family-centered communication to convey our interest in the concerns of the child and family. (Greet the family, for example, by introducing yourself and calling each family member by name.)

During the health interview, consider how best to ask questions and provide information in a way that will foster the elements of trust, respect, and empathy in order to establish a foundation for partnership. For example, you might incorporate social talk in the beginning of the health interview and allow Ms. Montes to state her questions or concerns before you begin to ask questions.

Step 2: Identify the Health Issues or Concerns Through Active Listening and "Fact-Finding"

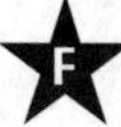

*Communication skills are critical to effective partnering with children and families. Some of these skills are covered in depth in the Communication module. The **Communication: Fostering Family-Centered Communication** handout from that module is an excellent supplement to this exercise.*

Begin by asking selected interview questions that are affirming and culturally sensitive. Start with open-ended questions, then follow up with specific questions. (The Bright Futures pocket guide provides a range of general health supervision questions for all ages, as well as age-specific questions for each recommended health visit. See References section.)

Part of this process involves communicating to the family what you think you've heard, then providing feedback and seeking clarification as needed.

As child health professionals, you consider the situation of the Montes family and decide that the central theme of the case is the mother's need to stay connected and thus reduce her isolation. In that way, she expects to provide good care for her child. As you seek to build a relationship with the family, enhancing the support systems available to Ms. Montes appears to be a reasonable short-term and long-term goal. To foster this goal, what questions would you want to ask the mother?

On the display board, the facilitator lists the learners' suggestions. Possible responses might include the following interview questions:

▶ What language would you like us to speak?

▶ Would you like me to arrange for an interpreter each time you come to see me?

▶ What was your life like in your country (or previous city)?

▶ How have you found moving to the city?

▶ Tell me about your neighborhood. [If appropriate, follow with: Do you feel safe there?]

▶ How do you and Moses like living with your brother?

▶ How is it to be a first-time mother?

▶ What specific things would you like to talk about today?

▶ What questions or concerns do you have about Moses' development or behavior?

▶ How would you describe Moses?

▶ Do you have friends in the city?

▶ What activities do you enjoy?

▶ Are you active in any religious or community groups?

▶ What do you and Moses enjoy together?

▶ Do other parents in your neighborhood enjoy some of the same activities as you?

▶ What are some of the main concerns in your life right now? How can I be of help to you?

How would you communicate to Ms. Montes your understanding of the issues that confront her? Build the questions in the exercise to address each identified concern. For example, questions that communicate your understanding might include the following:

▶ I know that moving to the city might not have been easy. What has been hardest for you?

▶ What things might help you in raising Moses?

▶ You said that you are worried about money.

• Please tell me a little more about your concern about money.

• Do you have medical insurance? What type is it?

• [If appropriate, ask also: Are you currently receiving WIC services, or food stamps?]

Step 3: Affirm the Strengths of the Child and Family

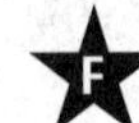 *This step is the most critical aspect of partnering and can never be overlooked. Omitting or missing this step can stall or even halt the process of building the partnership. The step consists of three stages: (1) identifying and affirming the child's and family's strengths so it is clear what each person brings to the partnership; (2) acknowledging and respecting each partner's contributions; and (3) commending the child and family for their specific health and developmental achievements.*

The facilitator then asks the learners:

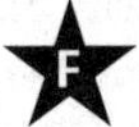 *What strengths of Ms. Montes can you identify?*

Possible responses might include the following:

▶ Ms. Montes clearly loves Moses and wants the best for him.

▶ Despite difficult circumstances, she has struggled hard to be a good mother to Moses.

▶ She asks many questions about Moses and seems very interested in his health and development.

▶ Although Ms. Montes' mother lives far away and her brother works long hours, her family obviously cares about her.

▶ Ms. Montes expresses a desire to work and to help provide a home for Moses.

The facilitator asks:

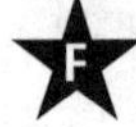 *How might you affirm the strengths of this family?*

Possible responses might include the following:

▶ Ask Ms. Montes to share some of the ways she has guided Moses' healthy development.

- Affirm that Ms. Montes knows her child best.
- Ask how she would describe Moses and what works best in soothing him when he cries. What kinds of games does he enjoy?
- Indicate that you recognize the strengths of her family support.
- Ask which support systems have worked for her—and which have not.
- Ask what Ms. Montes would find most helpful (e.g., print materials in her language, if available; referrals to legal services; help in addressing child support issues; links with other parents in similar situations; formal support groups; access to Web sites for information).

Step 4: Identify shared goals.

 *Child health professionals need to actively promote partnership with the child, family, and community. In building the partnership, it is important to identify and summarize mutual goals for the healthy development of the child, and to provide links between stated goals, health issues facing the child and family, and available resources in the community. This process elicits support for the partnership, coupled with awareness of community resources (knowledge base).*

The facilitator then ask the learners:

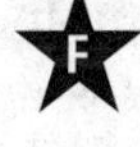 *What are some goals that you as the child health professional and Ms. Montes might share?*

Possible responses might include the following:

- Jointly identifying sources of support and social connections in the community.
- Developing strategies to help Ms. Montes gain more information and reassurance about health issues. For example, she can write down her questions as they arise and bring the list to the next health visit; the professional can provide written materials for her to take home, such as the Bright Futures Encounter Forms for Families (available in English and Spanish).
- Partnering to provide good health care information that meets the specific needs of the Montes family (not only providing important clinical guidance, but actively lis-

tening to and addressing concerns important to the Montes family).

- Nurturing Moses' growth and development by supporting the family's efforts to provide healthy nutrition and a safe home so Moses can achieve optimal health.

Step 5: Develop a joint plan of action based on stated goals.

The facilitator might introduce this step by asking the learners:

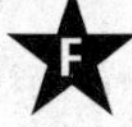 *Based on the mutual goals that have been identified, what might an action plan with the Montes family look like?*

(From our earlier case discussion, our proposed action plan should highlight strategies that will enhance support systems for Ms. Montes.)

Possible responses might include the following:

- The child health professional and Ms. Montes agree that she will write down her questions as they arise and bring them to the next health visit so the encounter can focus on the issues that are most important to her.
- The child health professional and Ms. Montes agree on one or two strategies to help strengthen her social and parenting support systems (e.g., participating in a parent support group, being active in her church group, reaching out to friends).
- The child health professional and Ms. Montes decide how best to communicate about issues that arise between appointments (e.g., telephone, e-mail, after-hours and emergency phone contacts).
- The child health professional provides referrals to WIC, social services, English for Speakers of Other Languages (ESOL) classes or other resources for families, local parent support groups.

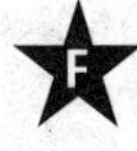 *Drawing on these suggestions, let's examine action plans in more detail. Effective action plans typically have the following characteristics:*

- Action plans are simple and achievable.
- Action plans have measurable goals and an identified timeline.

- Each partner has a role and responsibility in the plan.

- Each partner contributes to the development of the plan. Children, families, and communities who help develop the plan feel a greater sense of ownership and are more likely to follow through with the plan.

- The partners negotiate (using family-friendly negotiation skills) to ensure agreement on the plan.

- The plan builds in both a mechanism and a time for follow-up.

- The plan may also include advocacy to link families and resources as needed.

Step 6: Follow Up to Sustain the Partnership

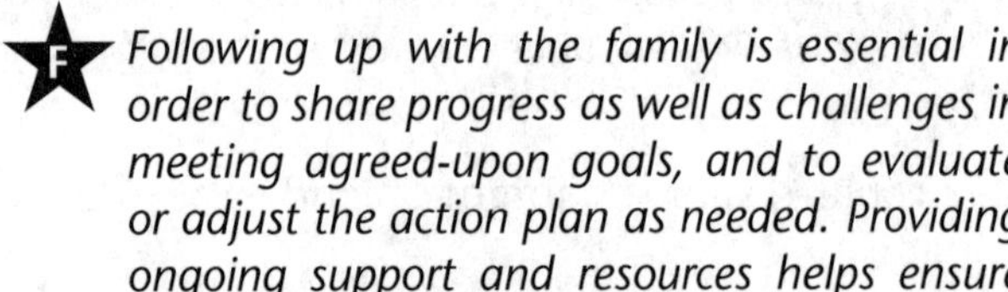 *Following up with the family is essential in order to share progress as well as challenges in meeting agreed-upon goals, and to evaluate or adjust the action plan as needed. Providing ongoing support and resources helps ensure the success of the action plan and the partnership.*

What are some ways that you as the child health professional could initiate follow-up with Ms. Montes?

Possible responses might include the following:

- Schedule a follow-up appointment with Ms. Montes before she leaves the office

- Provide daytime and after-hours phone numbers to Ms. Montes

- Be sure office staff at every level understand how important it is to facilitate easy access between the health care provider and the family, and to provide a timely response to the family's questions or concerns

- If specific action steps were identified, decide on a timeline for follow-up (e.g., Ms. Montes agrees to call the health professional in 2 weeks to discuss progress)

Final Discussion Point

In concluding the discussion, the facilitator asks the learners to reflect on and answer this question:

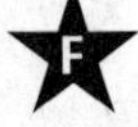 *How might outcomes differ for the Montes family when the health professional partners with Ms. Montes (versus not partnering)?*

Findings from National Survey of Parents

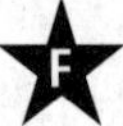 *As we conclude this session, I'm going to distribute the handout **On Listening**, which summarizes some valuable findings from a national survey of parents with young children.*

Take-Home Message

The facilitator summarizes by reading or paraphrasing the following:

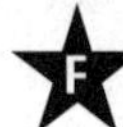 *In this session, we have identified six steps for effective partnering with children and families, and have practiced applying those steps through a case discussion. Partnering is a simple idea, but applying it can be quite complex, particularly in a clinical setting. The skills require practice and may take repeated efforts, even with the same child and family, before the partnership is formed. Remember that partnership development is a process and that partnerships fall along a continuum. Before we conclude, what questions remain about what we addressed today?*

Answers to the Guiding Questions

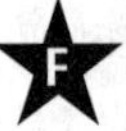 *Now that we have competed this session on Partnership, you should be able to answer the following questions:*

- How do open-ended and culturally sensitive interview questions facilitate communication between the child health professional and the family?

  - Open-ended and culturally sensitive interview questions can help start the conversation between the professional and the family, offer support and understanding, help the family identify areas of concern and set their agenda for the health visit, and promote joint problem-solving.

- How can child health professionals work in partnership with families to promote health, identify problems, and implement solutions?

  - Understanding the process of developing a partnership with a family, the steps involved, and the time and commitment needed to allow the development of a true partnership establishes a framework for interactions with families.

▶ What specific skills do child health professionals need in order to foster more effective partnerships with children, families, and/or communities?

  • The skills needed are active listening, fact-finding, demonstrating genuine interest in the child's health by taking time to understand the family's concerns, affirming their strengths, developing a mutually acceptable action plan, and following through with commitments made.

▶ Of the six steps for building partnerships, which step is most critical in building a partnership with the family?

  • Identifying and affirming the strengths of the child and family is the most critical step.

Evaluation

The facilitator now distributes the **Session Evaluation Form.** The facilitator also completes the **Facilitator Self-Assessment Form.**

Partnership: Session 2

PARTNERSHIP: BUILDING EFFECTIVE PARTNERSHIPS

A clinical partnership is a relationship in which participants join together to ensure health care delivery in a way that recognizes the critical roles and contributions of each partner (child, family, health professional, and community) in promoting health and preventing illness. Following are six steps for building effective health partnerships.

1. Model and encourage open, supportive communication with child and family.
- Integrate family-centered communication strategies
- Use communication skills to build trust, respect, and empathy

2. Identify health issues through active listening and "fact finding."
- Selectively choose Bright Futures general and age-appropriate interview questions
- Ask open-ended questions to encourage more complete sharing of information
- Communicate understanding of the issues and provide feedback

3. Affirm strengths of child and family.
- Recognize what each person brings to the partnership
- Acknowledge and respect each person's contributions
- Commend family for specific health and developmental achievements

4. Identify shared goals.
- Promote view of health supervision as partnership between child, family, health professional, and community
- Summarize mutual goals
- Provide links between stated goals, health issues, and available resources in community

5. Develop joint plan of action based on stated goals.
- Be sure that each partner has a role in developing the plan
- Keep plan simple and achievable
- Set measurable goals and specific timeline
- Use family-friendly negotiation skills to ensure agreement
- Build in mechanism and time for follow-up

6. Follow up: Sustaining the partnership.
- Share progress, successes, and challenges
- Evaluate and adjust plan
- Provide ongoing support and resources

Partnership: Session 2

CASE VIGNETTE:
THE MONTES FAMILY

Elise Montes, a 28-year-old woman, recently moved to the area and brings her 6-month-old baby, Moses, to your clinic for the first time. Born full term and healthy, Moses has had no medical problems and is developing well. As you interview Ms. Montes, you note that she is comfortably breastfeeding Moses and is responsive to his needs.

Ms. Montes' medical history indicates that she had a healthy pregnancy, although the circumstances were difficult. She is unmarried, and the baby's father left her after learning of her pregnancy. During the pregnancy, she sought shelter at a religious home that provides care for mothers and their infants. Ms. Montes' mother visited her briefly after Moses was born but has returned to her home in Venezuela.

Ms. Montes moved to the city to live with her brother. He is helpful with the baby when he is at home, but he works long hours. Ms. Montes says that she would like to get a job to help her brother with finances, because she worries a great deal about money.

Although Ms. Montes reports feeling tired frequently, she really enjoys Moses, especially now that he is starting to respond more. As you examine Moses, Ms. Montes asks several questions about his feeding, growth, and development. She says that she often thinks of questions at home but has difficulty remembering them once she arrives at the clinic.

Partnership: Session 2

CASE DISCUSSION: APPLYING THE SIX STEPS OF PARTNERSHIP

As you consider the case of Ms. Montes and Moses, think about the following areas:

- How would you encourage open and supportive communication with the mother?

- What questions could you ask to identify health issues in the family?

- How could you affirm this family's strengths?

- How will you communicate an understanding of the problem?

- What are the necessary resources that you and this mother need to be aware of? How might you begin to access these resources?

- What are the possible outcomes of this case? What are some of the action plans you and the mother might decide on together?

- How do the ethnicity and culture of this family or any family influence approaches to partnering?

Partnership: Session 2

ON LISTENING

The following information is based on findings from a national survey of parents with young children (Taaffe, Young, et al., 1998). Learners need to be particularly aware of the following issues when listening to families. Based on this survey, child health professionals may need to explore new interdisciplinary partnerships.

Most parents view the pediatric health care system as meeting the physical health needs of their young children; however, child health professionals often fail to discuss nonmedical questions with parents. Parents want more information and support on child-rearing concerns such as:

- Discipline
- Toilet training
- Responding to a crying baby
- Sleep patterns
- Newborn care
- Ways to encourage children to learn

Parents who receive comprehensive pediatric services and information report significantly higher levels of satisfaction with their child's provider. Services include:

- Home visit
- Packet of information on newborn
- Telephone advice line
- Booklet to track health status
- Checkup reminder system
- Developmental assessments

When meeting with families of young children, child health professionals need to be aware of these issues:

- Reading, singing, and showing affection are important influences on a child's cognitive and psychosocial development.
- Parents who speak with their physician or nurse about encouraging their child to learn are more likely to read to their child daily.
- Of the parents surveyed, 9% of mothers and 4% of fathers experienced three to five depressive symptoms at some time during the week before the survey; these

(continued on next page)

Partnership: Session 2

ON LISTENING (continued)

parents were more likely than parents without depressive symptoms to report frequent frustration with their child's behavior in a typical day ($p < 0.001$).

- Mothers were much more likely to breastfeed if a physician or nurse encouraged them to do so. Of the mothers surveyed, 74% who were encouraged to breastfeed actually did so, whereas only 45% of those who did not receive encouragement chose to breastfeed ($p < 0.001$).

Interventions by child health professionals have a positive effect on parental behaviors and health promotion in such areas as:

- Encouraging breastfeeding
- Encouraging reading
- Promoting wellness
- Addressing psychosocial concerns
- Individualizing anticipatory guidance
- Addressing parents' concerns on the perceived demands of their child to learn
- Finding creative ways to augment current services with the support of administrative and financial systems
- Recognizing the need for resources committed to preventive services
- Identifying creative solutions, including group well-child visits and a designated telephone line to discuss parental concerns about childhood behaviors

Reference

Taaffe, Young, Davis, K., Schoen, C., & Parker, S. (1998). Listening to parents: A national survey of parents with young children. *Archives of Pediatrics & Adolescent Medicine, 152,* 255–262. Copyright © 1998 American Medical Association. All rights reserved.

Partnership: Session 2

SESSION EVALUATION FORM

Session 2: Applying the Six Steps of Partnership

Date: _______________________________

Facilitator(s): _______________________________

Site: _______________________________

1. Overall, I found the "Applying the Six Steps of Partnership" session to be:

Not Useful			Very Useful	
1	2	3	4	5

2. The objectives of the session were:

Not Clear				Clear
1	2	3	4	5

3. The organization of the session was:

Poor				Excellent
1	2	3	4	5

4. The communication skills of the facilitator(s) were:

Poor				Excellent
1	2	3	4	5

5. The facilitator(s) stimulated interest in the subject matter:

Not at All			Very Much	
1	2	3	4	5

6. The facilitator(s) encouraged group participation:

Not at All			Very Much	
1	2	3	4	5

7. Handouts or visual aids (if used) were:

Not Helpful		Very Helpful		
1	2	3	4	5

8. Any additional comments?

____

____

____

9. The most useful features of the session were:

____

____

____

10. Suggestions for improvement

____

____

____

11. Suggestions for topics related to this session

____

____

____

Partnership: Session 2

FACILITATOR SELF-ASSESSMENT FORM

Directions: Please rate yourself from 1 to 5 on the following facilitator skills. The closer you are to a 5 within each domain, the more skilled you are at facilitation. We encourage you to complete this form prior to and after each teaching experience (e.g., a single session or an entire module). This will allow you to assess your performance as a facilitator over time.

Facilitator Behavior	1	2	3	4	5
Remains neutral					
Does not judge ideas					
Keeps the group focused on common task					
Asks clarifying questions					
Creates a climate free of criticism					
Encourages participation					
Structures participation					

Source: Adapted with permission from Welch, M. (1999). *Teaching diversity and cultural competence in health care: A trainer's guide.* San Francisco, CA: Perspectives of Differences Diversity Training and Consultation for Health Professionals (PODSDT).

References

Courtney, R., Ballard, E., & Fauver, S. et al. (1996). The partnership model: Working with individuals, families, and communities toward a new vision of health. *Public Health Nursing, 13*(30), 177–186.

Garfunkel, L.C. et al. (1998). Resident and family continuity in pediatric continuity clinic: Nine years of observation. *Pediatrics, 101,* 37–42.

Green, M., & Palfrey, J.S. (Eds.) (2002). *Bright futures: Guidelines for health supervision of infants, children, and adolescents* (2nd ed., rev.). Arlington, VA; National Center for Education in Maternal and Child Health.

Green, M., Palfrey, J.S., Clark, E.M., & Anastasi, J.M. (Eds.) (2002). *Bright futures: Guidelines for health supervision of infants, children, and adolescents* (2nd ed., rev.)—*Pocket guide.* Arlington, VA: National Center for Education in Maternal and Child Health.

Laraque, D., Barlow, B., Davidson, L., & Welborn, C. (1994). The Central Harlem Playground Injury Project: A model for change. *American Journal of Public Health, 84*(10), 1691–1692.

Taaffe, Young K., Davis, K., Schoen, C., & Parker, S. (1998). Listening to parents: A national survey of parents with young children. *Archives of Pediatric and Adolescent Medicine, 152,* 255–262.

Worchell, F.F., Prevatt, B.C., & Miner, J. et al. (1995). Pediatrician's communication style: Relationship to parent's perceptions and behaviors. *Journal of Pediatric Psychology, 20*(5), 633–644.

Resources

Benjamin, J.T., Cimino, S.A., & Hafler, J.P., Bright Futures Health Promotion Work Group, & Bernstein, H.H. 2002. The office visit: A time to promote health—but how? *Contemporary Pediatrics, 19*(2), 90–107.

Bonfield, A. [prod.] (2000). *Bright futures: Health supervision of infants, children, and adolescents* [videotape, part of the *Pediatrics in Practice* health promotion curriculum]. Sharon, MA: Biomedical Video and Multimedia.

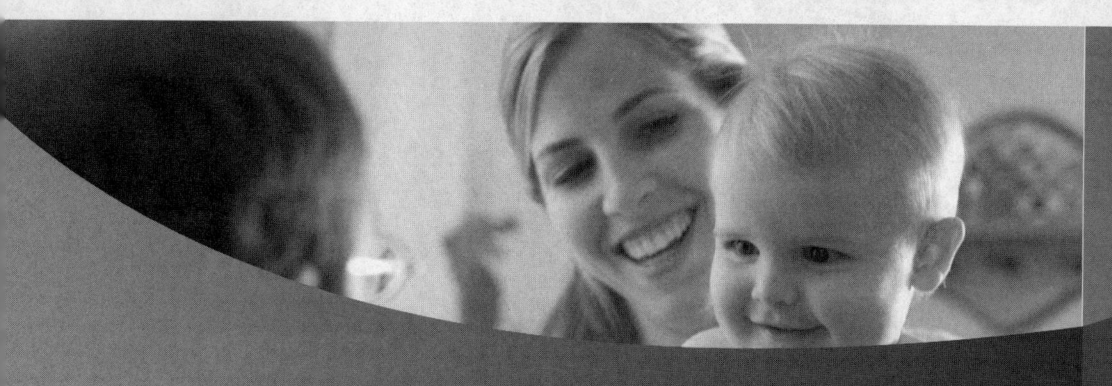

Chapter 4

Communication

Fostering Family-Centered Communication

Theodore C. Sectish

Gregory S. Blaschke

CONTENTS

Pediatrics in Practice

SESSION 2 (NONVIDEO OPTION): ELICITING THE CONCERNS OF CHILDREN AND FAMILIES

SESSION 3: INDIVIDUAL AND GROUP ASSESSMENT

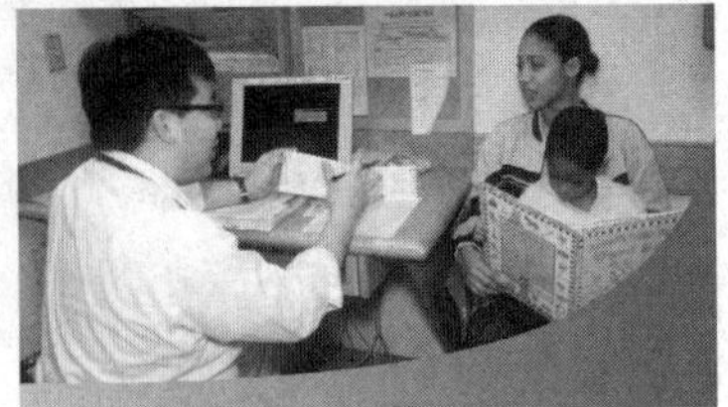

COMMUNICATION
Fostering Family-Centered Communication

OVERVIEW

Background

Family satisfaction with health care is closely related to the child health professional's ability to listen to and communicate with the child and family. Unfortunately, families often report unmet health care needs. A child health professional's skills in communication—particularly active listening—increase the prospect that a family's needs and concerns will be heard and addressed. Active listening involves listening for content and meaning, responding to the feelings expressed by children and their families, and noting carefully all verbal and nonverbal cues. Bright Futures emphasizes this approach with the use of interview questions to promote communication and clarify the family's concerns. Effective communication is especially important in our current practice environment where time is at a premium. By facilitating communication, child health professionals can help ensure that the needs and concerns of the child and family are met and that relevant information is provided.

Goal

The overall goal of this module is to enhance communication among child health professionals, children, and families during health visits by helping health professionals develop the skills, knowledge, and attitudes they need to communicate effectively.

This module will enable learners to:

▶ Listen actively

▶ Elicit the needs and concerns of children and families

▶ Acquire skills and practice in providing individual guidance

▶ Explore methods of assessing communication skills

Instructional Design

This module consists of three 30-minute sessions.

▶ Session 1 provides learners with the opportunity to improve their communication skills by learning to listen actively.

▶ Session 2 illustrates effective methods for eliciting the concerns and needs of children and their families and also provides learners with the opportunity to improve their communication skills.

▶ Each of the two sessions can be used as a separate, stand-alone offering, or the sessions can be combined. See the Facilitator's Guide for information on combining sessions.

▶ Each session has two distinct options—either the Video Option or the Nonvideo Option. The option chosen for presentation may be determined by considerations related to logistics, the equipment required, or the facilitation method preferred. For consistency, using the same option for both Session 1 and Session 2 is recommended.

▶ Session 3 can be used with either the Video Option or the Nonvideo Option.

▶ If a series covering three sessions is planned, there should be sufficient time between the sessions to allow for completion of any group projects or for self-assessment and review of skills in a practice setting.

Teaching Strategies

The teaching strategies used in this module include buzz groups, mini-presentation, role play (optional), and reflective exercise. These strategies have been selected to help learners develop the skills required to communicate effectively with children, parents, and their families. Please refer to the Facilitator's Guide for more information related to each strategy.

Evaluation

Learners will complete a **Session Evaluation Form** following each session and a **Module Evaluation Form** following the completion of the last session. Facilitators are encouraged to complete a **Facilitator Self-Assessment Form** prior to and following each teaching experience (e.g., a single session or an entire module) in order to assess their performance over time.

Guiding Questions

Learners who have completed the entire Communication module should be able to answer the following questions.

- ▶ What can I do to promote an atmosphere of trust so that children and families will share their true concerns?
- ▶ How can I incorporate the context of the family (community, school, cultural background) while providing comprehensive health care?
- ▶ How do I demonstrate that I am actively listening to my patients?
- ▶ How can I facilitate discussion during health visits with children and families?
- ▶ How do I determine the needs and concerns of children and families?
- ▶ What can I do to ensure that families leave the health visit with a feeling of confidence and a belief that their child's health care needs have been met?

INTRODUCTION TO TEACHING SESSIONS

Session 1 (Video and Nonvideo Options): Learning to Listen Actively

Objective (Video and Nonvideo Options)

The objective for this session is for the facilitator to:

- ▶ Provide learners with the opportunity to improve their communication skills by learning to listen actively

Materials

The materials and teaching aids needed for this session are:

Video Option

Handouts

- ▶ Communication: Fostering Family-Centered Communication
- ▶ Session Evaluation Form

Facilitator Form

- ▶ Facilitator Self-Assessment Form

Teaching Aids

- ▶ VCR and monitor
- ▶ Videotape of *The Doctor*
- ▶ 3" x 5" index cards
- ▶ Display board, flip chart, or chalkboard
- ▶ Markers or chalk

Nonvideo Option

Handouts

- ▶ Communication: Fostering Family-Centered Communication
- ▶ Session Evaluation Form

Facilitator Form

- ▶ Facilitator Self-Assessment Form

Teaching Aids

- ▶ 3" x 5" index cards
- ▶ Display board, flip chart, or chalkboard
- ▶ Markers or chalk

Time (Video and Nonvideo Options)

The time allocated for each version of this session is 30 minutes.

Session 2 (Video and Nonvideo Options): Eliciting the Concerns of Children and Families

Objectives (Video and Nonvideo Options)

The objectives for this session are for the facilitator to:

▶ Illustrate effective methods for eliciting the concerns and needs of children and their families

▶ Provide learners with the opportunity to improve their communication skills

Materials

The materials and teaching aids needed for this session are:

Video Option

Handouts

▶ Communication: Fostering Family-Centered Communication

▶ Session Evaluation Form

Facilitator Form

▶ Facilitator Self-Assessment Form

Teaching Aids

▶ VCR and monitor

▶ Videotape of *The Doctor*

▶ 3" x 5" index cards

▶ Display board, flip chart, or chalkboard

▶ Markers or chalk

Nonvideo Option

Handouts

▶ Communication: Fostering Family-Centered Communication

▶ Session Evaluation Form

Facilitator Form

▶ Facilitator Self-Assessment Form

Teaching Aids

▶ 3" x 5" index cards

▶ Display board, flip chart, or chalkboard

▶ Markers or chalk

Time (Video and Nonvideo Options)

The time allocated for each version of this session is 30 minutes.

Session 3: Individual and Group Assessment

Objective

The objectives for this session are for the facilitator to:

▶ Acquaint learners with communication evaluation methods including self-assessment, preceptor observation, group assessment, and patient-family survey

▶ Provide learners with opportunities to evaluate their communication skills

Materials

The materials and teaching aids needed for this session are:

Handouts

▶ Communication: Fostering Family-Centered Communication

▶ Learner Self-Assessment

▶ Preceptor Structured Observation Form

▶ Patient and Family Survey Form

▶ Session Evaluation Form

▶ Module Evaluation Form

Facilitator Form

▶ Facilitator Self-Assessment Form

Teaching Aids

▶ Display board, flip chart, or chalkboard

▶ Markers or chalk

Time

The time allocated for this session is 30 minutes.

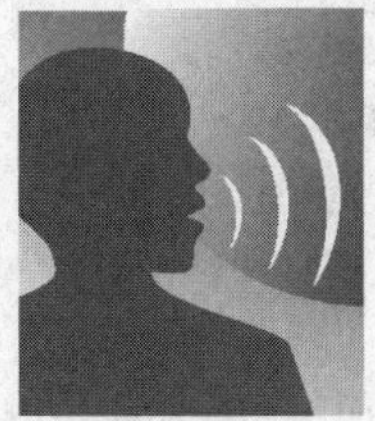

SESSION 1 (VIDEO OPTION):
Learning to Listen Actively

At the beginning of the session, the facilitator and learners should introduce themselves briefly. Ideas for creative introductions can be found in the Facilitator's Guide.

Setting the Context: The Bright Futures Concept

The facilitator **(F)** introduces the learners to the Bright Futures concept of health by reading or paraphrasing the following:

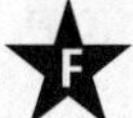 *The World Health Organization has defined health as "a state of complete physical, mental and social well-being and not merely the absence of disease or infirmity." Bright Futures embraces this broad definition of health—one that includes not only prevention of morbidity and mortality, but also the achievement of a child's full potential. In the Bright Futures concept of health, providing the capacity for healthy child development is as important as ameliorating illness or injury. Recognizing and acknowledging the strengths and resources of the child, family, and community are essential to promoting healthy growth and development.*

To build that capacity, the Pediatrics in Practice curriculum focuses on six core concepts: Partnership, Communication, Health Promotion/Illness Prevention, Time Management, Education, and Advocacy. The curriculum also includes a companion module (Health) and videotape that present an overview of Pediatrics in Practice and the Bright Futures approach.

Introducing the Session

Before introducing the session, the facilitator distributes the handout **Communication: Fostering Family-Centered Communication** to the learners.

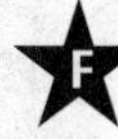 *Today's session is the first of three that comprise the* Pediatrics in Practice *Communication module.*

This session focuses on active listening skills. Family satisfaction with health care is closely related to the child health professional's ability to listen to and communicate with the child and family.

Skills in communication, particularly active listening, increase the pediatric provider's ability to hear and address the needs and concerns of children and their families. Active listening involves listening for content and meaning, responding to the feelings expressed, and carefully noting verbal and nonverbal cues.

Effective communication is especially important in our current practice environment where time is at a premium. By facilitating communication, child health professionals can help ensure that the needs and concerns of the child and family are met and that relevant information is provided.

In today's session, our objectives will be to:

▶ *Focus on and discuss the key elements of active listening*

▶ *View a videotape segment that illustrates the importance of listening actively in order to build a trusting partnership with children and families*

▶ *Reflect on patient- or family-centered communication as depicted in the videotape scenario*

When we have completed the session, you should be able to answer the following questions:

▶ *What can I do to promote an atmosphere of trust so that children and families will share their true concerns?*

▶ *How can I incorporate the context of the family (community, school, cultural background) while providing comprehensive health care?*

How do I demonstrate that I am actively listening to my patients?

Discussion and Exercises

Videotape Stimulus and Reflection

[Note to facilitator on setting up the VCR: The relevant scenes from the movie *The Doctor* follow the Bright Futures video used in the Health module.]

The facilitator introduces the videotape segment from the movie *The Doctor*.

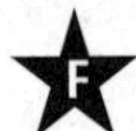
In the movie The Doctor, *William Hurt portrays a physician whose own illness forces him to assume the role of a patient. The experience provides him with personal insight about the importance of communicating effectively with patients.*

This segment of the film demonstrates a patient- or family-centered communication style. In this clip, the physician is meeting with a male patient before surgery. His interaction with the patient serves as an example for your reflection.

After the videotape segment has been viewed, the facilitator guides the learners through the following reflective exercise:

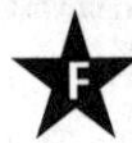
For the next 3 minutes, I would like each of you to think about the videotape segment you have just watched. During this reflective time, slowly narrow your focus and concentrate on the positive and negative aspects of the health professional's listening skills. What worked well? What did not work as well?

Distribute 3" x 5" index cards for those who find jotting a few notes helpful. Allow 3 minutes for reflection without interruption.

After the 3 minutes of reflection, the facilitator initiates a "buzz group" discussion.

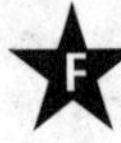
Now turn to the person sitting beside you and discuss your thoughts about the health professional's communication skills as fully as possible in the next 2 minutes.

The facilitator writes these questions on a display board or flip chart and says:

Try to address the following questions directly or indirectly in your discussion:

- *What words, behaviors, questions, or mannerisms were used?*
- *What aspects of the interview contributed to improved communication?*

- *What elements of the physician's communication were most effective?*
- *How did active listening increase the effectiveness of the physician's communication style?*
- *Did anything make the segment powerful or illustrative?*

After the discussion period, the facilitator asks:

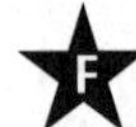
Who would like to describe their thoughts and reactions?

Discussion Questions

The facilitator continues the discussion and encourages all learners to offer their ideas.

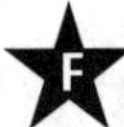
What elements of active listening contribute to improved communication and interactions among child health professionals, children, and families?

Using a display board or flip chart, the facilitator records the observations and suggestions made by the learners.

Examples:

Active listening:

- Is patient or family centered, not provider centered
- Involves both verbal and nonverbal elements of communication
- Will elicit the concerns and needs of children and families
- Promotes satisfaction, trust, and partnership

The facilitator continues with a discussion of the use of active listening skills in establishing rapport and building trust with children and families.

What observations have you made about the use of active listening skills in establishing rapport and building trust with children and families?

Once again the facilitator records the learners' responses.

Examples:

The pediatric provider establishes rapport and builds trust by:

- Listening for content and meaning
- Asking about the child and family's feelings and responding to the feelings they express

▶ Offering supportive comments

▶ Noting all verbal and nonverbal cues carefully

 *The nuances of the health interview are complex. However, child health professionals who use active listening as a regular part of their communication with children and families are more likely to make important observations about how well they are establishing rapport and building trust.*

How do active listening skills help to focus a health interview?

Examples:

Active listening allows the pediatric provider to:

▶ Address the important issues that children and families bring to the health visit

▶ Clarify statements with follow-up questions

▶ Offer information or explanations

Take-Home Message

The facilitator ends the session with the following:

 *Child health professionals who are both effective and time efficient use active listening skills to promote partnership, improve family satisfaction, and build trust with children and their families. Active listening requires the pediatric provider to listen for content and meaning.*

The facilitator asks the learners to refer to the **Communication: Fostering Family-Centered Communication** handout and says:

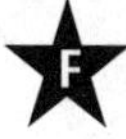 *This handout highlights both verbal and nonverbal behaviors that promote active listening during a health visit. It identifies behaviors that create a welcoming environment for open communication and help to elicit the needs and concerns of children and their families. Please take some time before our next session to review this information and reflect on it. Before we conclude, what questions remain about what we addressed today?*

Answers to the Guiding Questions

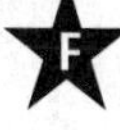 *Now that we have completed this session on Communication, you should be able to answer the following questions:*

▶ What can I do to promote an atmosphere of trust so that children and families will share their true concerns?

• Listen for content and meaning

• Ask about child and family's feelings and respond to the feelings they express

• Offer supportive comments

• Note all verbal and nonverbal cues carefully

▶ How can I incorporate the context of the family (community, school, cultural background) while providing comprehensive health care?

• Use family-centered communication skills

• Discuss family life, community, and school

▶ How do I demonstrate that I am actively listening to my patients?

• Allow children and their families to state concerns without interruption

• Address the important issues that children and families bring to the health visit

• Clarify statements with follow-up questions

Planning for the Next Session (if Session 2 is planned)

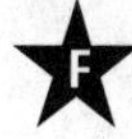 *In the next session, which focuses on eliciting the concerns of children and families, we will continue our discussion of effective communication methods.*

Please take some time before the next session to reflect on how you would encourage children and families to verbalize or otherwise indicate their expectations for the health visit.

(For those programs using a 2-hour workshop format, this could serve as a breakpoint and allow time for reflection.)

Evaluation

The facilitator now distributes the **Session Evaluation Form.** The facilitator also completes the **Facilitator Self-Assessment Form.**

Communication: Session 1

COMMUNICATION: FOSTERING FAMILY-CENTERED COMMUNICATION

Effective Behaviors
- Greet each family member and introduce self
- Use names of family members
- Incorporate social talk in the beginning of the interview
- Show interest and attention
- Demonstrate empathy
- Appear patient and unhurried
- Acknowledge concerns, fears, and feelings of child and family
- Use ordinary language, not medical jargon
- Use Bright Futures general and age-appropriate interview questions
- Give information clearly
- Query level of understanding and allow sufficient time for response
- Encourage additional questions
- Discuss family life, community, school

Active Listening Skills: Verbal Behaviors
- Allow child and parents to state concerns without interruption
- Encourage questions and answer them completely
- Clarify statements with follow-up questions
- Ask about feelings
- Acknowledge stress or difficulties
- Allow sufficient time for a response (wait time >3 seconds)
- Offer supportive comments
- Restate in the parent's or child's words
- Offer information or explanations

Active Listening Skills: Nonverbal Behaviors
- Nod in agreement
- Sit down at the level of the child and make eye contact
- Interact with or play with the child
- Show expression, attention, concern, or interest
- Convey understanding and empathy
- Touch child or parent (if appropriate)
- Draw pictures to clarify
- Demonstrate techniques

Source: Reproduced with permission from Green, M., Palfrey, J.S., Clark, E.M., & Anastasi, J.M. (Eds.) (2002). *Bright futures: Guidelines for health supervision of infants, children, and adolescents* (2nd ed., rev.)—*Pocket guide.* Arlington, VA: National Center for Education in Maternal and Child Health.

Communication: Session 1

SESSION EVALUATION FORM

Session 1: Learning to Listen Actively

Date: ___________________________

Facilitator(s): _______________________________________

Site: ____

---

1. Overall, I found the "Learning to Listen Actively" session to be:

Not Useful			Very Useful	
1	2	3	4	5

2. The objectives of the session were:

Not Clear				Clear
1	2	3	4	5

3. The organization of the session was:

Poor			Excellent	
1	2	3	4	5

4. The communication skills of the facilitator(s) were:

Poor			Excellent	
1	2	3	4	5

5. The facilitator(s) stimulated interest in the subject matter:

Not at All			Very Much	
1	2	3	4	5

6. The facilitator(s) encouraged group participation:

Not at All			Very Much	
1	2	3	4	5

7. Handouts or visual aids (if used) were:

Not Helpful		Very Helpful	
1	2	3	4	5

8. Any additional comments?

   ____
   ____
   ____

9. The most useful features of the session were:

   ____
   ____
   ____

10. Suggestions for improvement

   ____
   ____
   ____

11. Suggestions for topics related to this session

   ____
   ____
   ____

Communication: Session 1

FACILITATOR SELF-ASSESSMENT FORM

Directions: Please rate yourself from 1 to 5 on the following facilitator skills. The closer you are to a 5 within each domain, the more skilled you are at facilitation. We encourage you to complete this form prior to and after each teaching experience (e.g., a single session or an entire module). This will allow you to assess your performance as a facilitator over time.

Facilitator Behavior	1	2	3	4	5
Remains neutral					
Does not judge ideas					
Keeps the group focused on common task					
Asks clarifying questions					
Creates a climate free of criticism					
Encourages participation					
Structures participation					

Source: Adapted with permission from Welch, M. (1999). *Teaching diversity and cultural competence in health care: A trainer's guide.* San Francisco, CA: Perspectives of Differences Diversity Training and Consultation for Health Professionals (PODSDT).

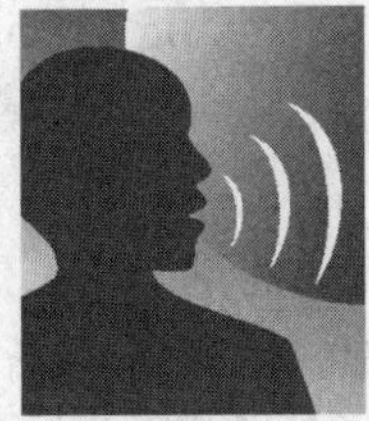

SESSION 1 (NONVIDEO OPTION):
Learning to Listen Actively

At the beginning of the session, the facilitator and learners should introduce themselves briefly. Ideas for creative introductions can be found in the Facilitator's Guide.

Setting the Context: The Bright Futures Concept

The facilitator **(F)** introduces the learners to the Bright Futures concept of health by reading or paraphrasing the following:

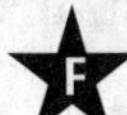 *The World Health Organization has defined health as "a state of complete physical, mental and social well-being and not merely the absence of disease or infirmity." Bright Futures embraces this broad definition of health—one that includes not only prevention of morbidity and mortality, but also the achievement of a child's full potential. In the Bright Futures concept of health, providing the capacity for healthy child development is as important as ameliorating illness or injury. Recognizing and acknowledging the strengths and resources of the child, family, and community are essential to promoting healthy growth and development.*

To build that capacity, the Pediatrics in Practice curriculum focuses on six core concepts: Partnership, Communication, Health Promotion/Illness Prevention, Time Management, Education, and Advocacy. The curriculum also includes a companion module (Health) and videotape that present an overview of Pediatrics in Practice and the Bright Futures approach.

Introducing the Session

Before introducing the session, the facilitator distributes the handout Communication: Fostering Family-Centered Communication to the learners.

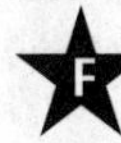 *Today's session is the first of three that comprise the* Pediatrics in Practice *Communication module.*

This session focuses on active listening skills. Family satisfaction with health care is closely related to the child health professional's ability to listen to and communicate with the child and family.

Skills in communication, particularly active listening, increase the pediatric provider's ability to recognize and address the needs and concerns of children and their families. Active listening involves listening for content and meaning, responding to the feelings expressed, and carefully noting verbal and nonverbal cues.

Effective communication is especially important in our current practice environment where time is at a premium. By facilitating communication, child health professionals can help ensure that the needs and concerns of the child and family are met and that relevant information is provided.

In today's session, our objectives will be to:

▶ *Focus on and discuss the key elements of active listening*

▶ *Complete a reflective exercise on the use of active listening to build a trusting partnership with children and families*

When we have completed the session, you should be able to answer the following questions:

▶ *What can I do to promote an atmosphere of trust so that children and families will share their true concerns?*

▶ *How can I incorporate the context of the family (community, school, cultural background) while providing comprehensive health care?*

▶ *How do I demonstrate that I am actively listening to my patients?*

Discussion and Exercises

Reflective Exercise

The facilitator describes the reflective exercise:

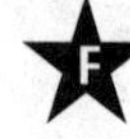 *I would like each of you to spend 3 minutes considering the many health encounters you have observed or experienced personally over the last year. Think of the various settings in which you interact with children and families or observe interactions among pediatric providers and families.*

Slowly narrow your focus and concentrate on recreating one specific experience that stands out as particularly powerful. For example, do you remember a time when the real concerns of the family were missed, or when effective listening led to a meaningful discussion or disclosure?

> ▶ *What were the positive and the negative aspects of the child health professional's or your listening skills?*
>
> ▶ *What worked well? What did not work as well?*

The facilitator distributes 3" x 5" index cards for those who find jotting a few notes helpful and allows 3 minutes for reflection without interruption.

After the 3 minutes of reflection, the facilitator initiates a "buzz group" discussion (people in small groups talking together around a particular focus):

 *Now turn to the person sitting beside you and describe your experience as fully as possible in the next 2 minutes.*

The facilitator writes these questions on a display board or flip chart and says:

 *Try to address the following questions directly or indirectly as your story unfolds:*

> ▶ *In what context did this experience occur?*
>
> ▶ *What words, behaviors, questions, or mannerisms were used?*
>
> ▶ *What aspects of the interview or encounter contributed to or could have contributed to improved communication?*
>
> ▶ *Was the communication centered on the child and family or on the provider?*
>
> ▶ *What active listening skills were demonstrated in the encounter?*
>
> ▶ *Were important family needs or concerns missed? Or were they identified?*

> ▶ *What do you feel made your example powerful and illustrative?*
>
> ▶ *How have you changed personally and professionally as a result of the experience?*
>
> ▶ *What will you do differently or improve upon in your future practice as a result of the experience?*

After the discussion period, the facilitator asks:

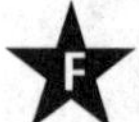 *Who would like to describe and discuss their experience?*

Discussion Questions

The facilitator continues the discussion and encourages all learners to offer their ideas.

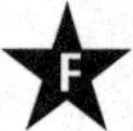 *What elements of active listening contribute to improved communication and interactions among child health professionals, children, and families?*

Using a display board or flip chart, the facilitator records the observations and suggestions made by the learners.

Examples:

Active listening:

> ▶ Is patient or family centered, not provider centered
>
> ▶ Involves both verbal and nonverbal elements of communication
>
> ▶ Will elicit the concerns and needs of children and families
>
> ▶ Promotes satisfaction, trust, and partnership

The facilitator continues with a discussion of the use of active listening skills in establishing rapport and building trust with children and families.

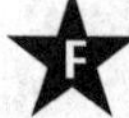 *What observations have you made about the use of active listening skills in establishing rapport and building trust with children and families?*

Once again the facilitator records the learners' responses.

Examples:

The pediatric provider establishes rapport and builds trust by:

> ▶ Listening for content and meaning
>
> ▶ Asking about the child and family's feelings and responding to the feelings they express

▶ Offering supportive comments

▶ Noting all verbal and nonverbal cues carefully

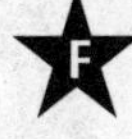 *The nuances of the health interview are complex. However, child health professionals who use active listening as a regular part of their communication with children and families are more likely to make important observations about how well they are establishing rapport and building trust.*

How do active listening skills help to focus a health interview?

Examples:

Active listening allows the pediatric provider to:

▶ Address the important issues that children and families bring to the health visit

▶ Clarify statements with follow-up questions

▶ Offer information or explanations

Take-Home Message

The facilitator ends the session with the following:

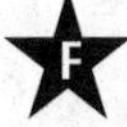 *Child health professionals who are both effective and time-efficient use active listening skills to promote partnership, improve family satisfaction, and build trust with children and their families. Active listening requires the pediatric provider to listen for content and meaning.*

The facilitator asks the learners to refer to the **Communication: Fostering Family-Centered Communication** handout and says:

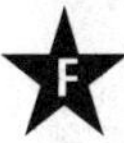 *This handout highlights both verbal and nonverbal behaviors that promote active listening during a health visit. It identifies behaviors that create a welcoming environment for open communication and help to elicit the needs and concerns of children and their families. Please take some time before our next session to review this information and reflect on it. Before we conclude, what questions remain about what we addressed today?*

Answers to the Guiding Questions

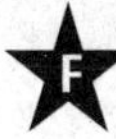 *Now that we have completed this session on Communication, you should be able to answer the following questions:*

▶ What can I do to promote an atmosphere of trust so that children and families will share their true concerns?

● Listen for content and meaning

● Ask about child and family's feelings and respond to the feelings they express

● Offer supportive comments

● Note all verbal and nonverbal cues carefully

▶ How can I incorporate the context of the family (community, school, cultural background) while providing comprehensive health care?

● Use family-centered communication skills

● Discuss family life, community, and school

▶ How do I demonstrate that I am actively listening to my patients?

● Allow children and their families to state concerns without interruption

● Address the important issues that children and families bring to the health visit

● Clarify statements with follow-up questions

Planning for the Next Session (if Session 2 is planned)

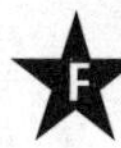 *In the next session, which focuses on eliciting the concerns of children and families, we will continue our discussion of effective communication methods.*

Please take some time before the next session to reflect on how you would encourage children and families to verbalize or otherwise indicate their expectations for the health visit.

(For those programs using a 2-hour workshop format, this could serve as a breakpoint and allow time for reflection.)

Evaluation

The facilitator now distributes the **Session Evaluation Form**. The facilitator also completes the **Facilitator Self-Assessment Form**.

Communication: Session 1

COMMUNICATION: FOSTERING FAMILY-CENTERED COMMUNICATION

Effective Behaviors
- Greet each family member and introduce self
- Use names of family members
- Incorporate social talk in the beginning of the interview
- Show interest and attention
- Demonstrate empathy
- Appear patient and unhurried
- Acknowledge concerns, fears, and feelings of child and family
- Use ordinary language, not medical jargon
- Use Bright Futures general and age-appropriate interview questions
- Give information clearly
- Query level of understanding and allow sufficient time for response
- Encourage additional questions
- Discuss family life, community, school

Active Listening Skills: Verbal Behaviors
- Allow child and parents to state concerns without interruption
- Encourage questions and answer them completely
- Clarify statements with follow-up questions
- Ask about feelings
- Acknowledge stress or difficulties
- Allow sufficient time for a response (wait time >3 seconds)
- Offer supportive comments
- Restate in the parent's or child's words
- Offer information or explanations

Active Listening Skills: Nonverbal Behaviors
- Nod in agreement
- Sit down at the level of the child and make eye contact
- Interact with or play with the child
- Show expression, attention, concern, or interest
- Convey understanding and empathy
- Touch child or parent (if appropriate)
- Draw pictures to clarify
- Demonstrate techniques

Communication: Session 1

SESSION EVALUATION FORM

Session 1: Learning to Listen Actively

Date: _______________________________

Facilitator(s): _______________________________

Site: _______________________________

---

1. Overall, I found the "Learning to Listen Actively" session to be:

Not Useful			Very Useful	
1	2	3	4	5

2. The objectives of the session were:

Not Clear				Clear
1	2	3	4	5

3. The organization of the session was:

Poor			Excellent	
1	2	3	4	5

4. The communication skills of the facilitator(s) were:

Poor			Excellent	
1	2	3	4	5

5. The facilitator(s) stimulated interest in the subject matter:

Not at All			Very Much	
1	2	3	4	5

6. The facilitator(s) encouraged group participation:

Not at All			Very Much	
1	2	3	4	5

7. Handouts or visual aids (if used) were:

Not Helpful		Very Helpful		
1	2	3	4	5

8. Any additional comments?

   ____
   ____
   ____

9. The most useful features of the session were:

   ____
   ____
   ____

10. Suggestions for improvement

    ____
    ____
    ____

11. Suggestions for topics related to this session

    ____
    ____
    ____

Communication: Session 1

FACILITATOR SELF-ASSESSMENT FORM

Directions: Please rate yourself from 1 to 5 on the following facilitator skills. The closer you are to a 5 within each domain, the more skilled you are at facilitation. We encourage you to complete this form prior to and after each teaching experience (e.g., a single session or an entire module). This will allow you to assess your performance as a facilitator over time.

Facilitator Behavior	1	2	3	4	5
Remains neutral					
Does not judge ideas					
Keeps the group focused on common task					
Asks clarifying questions					
Creates a climate free of criticism					
Encourages participation					
Structures participation					

Source: Adapted with permission from Welch, M. (1999). *Teaching diversity and cultural competence in health care: A trainer's guide.* San Francisco, CA: Perspectives of Differences Diversity Training and Consultation for Health Professionals (PODSDT).

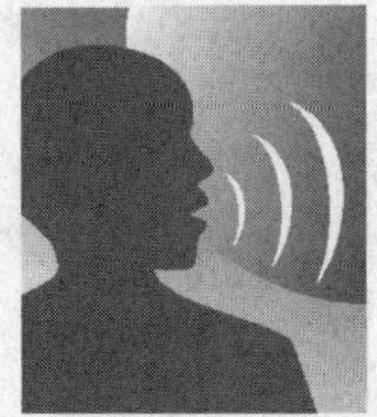

SESSION 2 (VIDEO OPTION):
Eliciting the Concerns of Children and Families

Session 2, Video Option, should be chosen if Video Option was used for Session 1.

At the beginning of the session, the facilitator and learners should introduce themselves briefly. (If the same group has recently completed Session 1, the facilitator may decide that introductions are not needed.) Ideas for creative introductions can be found in the Facilitator's Guide.

Setting the Context: The Bright Futures Concept

(May be omitted if recently presented or when sessions are combined.)

The facilitator **(F)** introduces the learners to the Bright Futures concept of health by reading or paraphrasing the following:

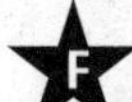 *The World Health Organization has defined health as "a state of complete physical, mental and social well-being and not merely the absence of disease or infirmity." Bright Futures embraces this broad definition of health—one that includes not only prevention of morbidity and mortality, but also the achievement of a child's full potential. In the Bright Futures concept of health, providing the capacity for healthy child development is as important as ameliorating illness or injury. Recognizing and acknowledging the strengths and resources of the child, family, and community are essential to promoting healthy growth and development.*

To build that capacity, the Pediatrics in Practice curriculum focuses on six core concepts: Partnership, Communication, Health Promotion/Illness Prevention, Time Manage ment, Education, and Advocacy. The curriculum also includes a companion module (Health) and videotape that present an overview of

Pediatrics in Practice and the Bright Futures approach.

Introducing the Session

Before introducing the session, the facilitator distributes the handout **Communication: Fostering Family-Centered Communication** to the learners. (The facilitator may choose not to distribute the handout if it was recently given to the same learners.)

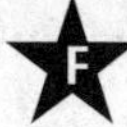 *Today's session is the second of three that comprise the* Pediatrics in Practice *Communication module.*

This session focuses on eliciting the needs and concerns of children and families. Family satisfaction with their health visit is intimately associated with the communication skills of the health professional. All too often, child health professionals do not elicit a family's important concerns. Children and their families leave their health visits with unmet needs. If a child or family feels that their concerns were not heard and addressed, the pediatric provider has lost the opportunity to provide comprehensive, quality health care and strengthen his or her relationship with the child and family.

Effective communication during health visits is essential to building trust and creating partnerships with children and families. Communication skills can be practiced and improved. Today we will view another videotape segment from the movie The Doctor and focus our attention on eliciting the concerns of children and families.

In today's session, our objectives will be to:

▶ *Focus on the communication skills required to elicit the needs and concerns of children and families*

▶ *View a videotape segment to initiate discussion on communication styles and on identifying family concerns*

▶ *Compare provider-centered and patient- or family-centered communication styles*

When we have completed the session, you should be able to answer the following questions:

▶ *How can I facilitate discussion during health visits with children and families?*

▶ *How do I determine the needs and concerns of children and families?*

▶ *What can I do to ensure that families leave the health visit with a feeling of confidence and a belief that their child's health care needs have been met?*

Discussion and Exercises

Videotape Stimulus and Reflection

[Note to facilitator on setting up the VCR: The relevant scenes from the movie *The Doctor* follow the Bright Futures video used in the Health module.]

The facilitator introduces the videotape segment from the movie *The Doctor*.

 *In the last session, we viewed a clip from the movie* The Doctor, *which illustrated patient- or family-centered communication. In this segment of the movie, an Ear, Nose, and Throat specialist examines the physician, portrayed by William Hurt. This clip illustrates the provider-centered communication style.*

After the videotape segment has been viewed, the facilitator guides the learners through the following reflective exercise:

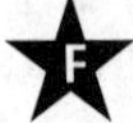 *For the next 3 minutes, I would like each of you to think about the videotape segment you have just watched. During this reflective time, slowly narrow your focus and concentrate on the communication style of the ENT specialist and on the needs and concerns of the patient. Make note of the words, behaviors, mannerisms, and questions that were used.*

Distribute 3" x 5" index cards for those who find jotting a few notes helpful; allow 3 minutes for reflection without interruption.

After the 3 minutes of reflection, the facilitator initiates a "buzz group" discussion (people in small groups talking together around a particular focus), as follows:

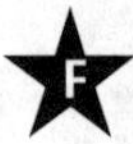 *Now turn to the person sitting beside you and describe your observations about the ENT specialist's communication skills as fully as possible in the next 2 minutes.*

The facilitator writes the following questions on a display board or flip chart and says:

 *Try to address these questions directly or indirectly as your observations unfold, pointing out both verbal and nonverbal aspects of communication:*

▶ *What methods did the ENT specialist use to elicit the concerns of the patient?*

▶ *What aspects of the interview contributed to poor communication?*

▶ *What was missing in this encounter?*

▶ *Did anything make the segment powerful or illustrative? If so, what?*

After the "buzz group" discussion period, the facilitator asks:

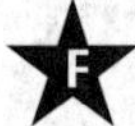 *Who would like to describe their observations?*

Discussion Questions and Answers

If discussion does not occur spontaneously or flow easily, the facilitator might consider the use of discussion questions. Ask only one question at a time.

 ▶ *What methods did this physician use to elicit the patient's concerns?*

The physician used a provider-centered approach to communication by controlling the interview, dominating the agenda, and using closed questions.

▶ *How successful was she in eliciting the concerns of the patient? Why?*

She focused on the task of gathering and giving information and kept the patient in a passive role. Although she inquired about his concerns, she did not acknowledge them. Nor did she inquire about his feelings, worries, or needs. Her task-oriented and business-like approach conveyed detachment and emotional distance.

▶ *What are your impressions about her communication style? Was her style effective or ineffective?*

While there are obvious shortcomings to her approach, she was effective in obtaining information, controlling the interview, and accomplishing her agenda. However, there was little time for discussion, no negotiation, nor any partnership.

In general, the provider-centered communication style limits the effectiveness of the health interview by neglecting or ignoring the concerns and needs of children and families.

The facilitator might continue with a discussion of communication styles in different circumstances.

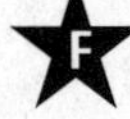

You might regard the style demonstrated in the scene as being typical of a surgeon, who would be likely to opt for a "provider-centered" approach. Yet, we all vary our personal style to adapt to the circumstances of the moment. We commonly experience communication challenges due to time pressures, the settings in which we practice, or our own biases or perceptions about the seriousness of a family's concerns.

During residency training, you often find yourself in a variety of circumstances. You may be post-call or pre-call, or you may be in specific clinical settings such as the ER, continuity clinic, or an intensive care unit.

▶ *Can you suggest some patient- or family-centered approaches to communication in these different circumstances?*

▶ *How would communication differ if patient- or family-centered methods (rather than provider-centered methods) were applied?*

The facilitator asks the learners to refer to the **Communication: Fostering Family-Centered Communication** handout.

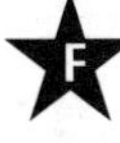

This sheet highlights behaviors that help determine a child or family's needs or concerns during a health encounter. Please take a moment to examine the list and identify specific behaviors that create a welcoming environment for open communication. You may want to reflect on asking open-ended questions and waiting for responses.

How much "wait time" do you provide in your encounters with children and families?

The facilitator continues:

Ideally, wait time should be at least 3 seconds following a question. This gives the child and family time to process the question. The wait may seem trivial, but if you actually observe child health professionals in their encounters with families and look for evidence of the 3-second wait time, you will appreciate just how long 3 seconds can be. Wait time is essential in accomplishing the goal of eliciting the concerns of children and families.

Take-Home Message

The facilitator ends the session with the following:

The ability to elicit the needs and concerns of children and their families is an essential communication skill in pediatric health care. By examining the shortcomings and disadvantages of provider-centered communication, we have seen clearly the effectiveness of patient- or family-centered communication. We have also explored the use of the 3-second wait time as a valuable tool in eliciting the true concerns of children and families. Before we conclude, what questions remain about what we addressed today?

Answers to the Guiding Questions

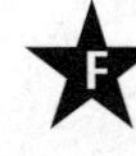

Now that we have completed this session on Communication, you should be able to answer the following questions:

▶ How can I facilitate discussion during health visits with children and families?

- Show interest and attention
- Appear patient and unhurried
- Use ordinary language, not medical jargon
- Encourage additional questions

▶ How do I determine the needs and concerns of children and families?

- Ask open-ended questions
- Wait at least 3 seconds for a response
- Ask follow-up questions

▶ What can I do to ensure that families leave the health visit with a feeling of confidence and a belief that their child's health care needs have been met?

- Encourage questions and answer them completely
- Give information clearly
- Draw pictures to clarify or demonstrate techniques

Planning for the Next Session (if Session 3 is planned)

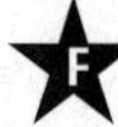 *In the next session, which focuses on evaluating communication skills, we will look at a variety of tools and forms that can assist you in assessing the effectiveness of your communication skills. As preparation for our next session, please think about some ways you might receive feedback from the children and families you encounter during health visits.*

(For those programs using a 2-hour workshop format, this could serve as a breakpoint and allow time for reflection.)

Evaluation

The facilitator now distributes the **Session Evaluation Form.** The facilitator also completes the **Facilitator Self-Assessment Form.**

Communication: Session 2

COMMUNICATION: FOSTERING FAMILY-CENTERED COMMUNICATION

Effective Behaviors

- Greet each family member and introduce self
- Use names of family members
- Incorporate social talk in the beginning of the interview
- Show interest and attention
- Demonstrate empathy
- Appear patient and unhurried
- Acknowledge concerns, fears, and feelings of child and family
- Use ordinary language, not medical jargon
- Use Bright Futures general and age-appropriate interview questions
- Give information clearly
- Query level of understanding and allow sufficient time for response
- Encourage additional questions
- Discuss family life, community, school

Active Listening Skills: Verbal Behaviors

- Allow child and parents to state concerns without interruption
- Encourage questions and answer them completely
- Clarify statements with follow-up questions
- Ask about feelings
- Acknowledge stress or difficulties
- Allow sufficient time for a response (wait time >3 seconds)
- Offer supportive comments
- Restate in the parent's or child's words
- Offer information or explanations

Active Listening Skills: Nonverbal Behaviors

- Nod in agreement
- Sit down at the level of the child and make eye contact
- Interact with or play with the child
- Show expression, attention, concern, or interest
- Convey understanding and empathy
- Touch child or parent (if appropriate)
- Draw pictures to clarify
- Demonstrate techniques

Source: Reproduced with permission from Green, M., Palfrey, J.S., Clark, E.M, & Anastasi, J.M. (Eds.) (2002). *Bright futures: Guidelines for health supervision of infants, children, and adolescents* (2nd ed., rev.)—*Pocket guide.* Arlington, VA: National Center for Education in Maternal and Child Health.

Communication: Session 2

SESSION EVALUATION FORM

Session 2: Eliciting the Concerns of Children and Families

Date: _______________________________

Facilitator(s): _______________________________

Site: _______________________________

---

1. Overall, I found the "Eliciting the Concerns of Children and Families" session to be:

Not Useful			Very Useful	
1	2	3	4	5

2. The objectives of the session were:

Not Clear				Clear
1	2	3	4	5

3. The organization of the session was:

Poor				Excellent
1	2	3	4	5

4. The communication skills of the facilitator(s) were:

Poor				Excellent
1	2	3	4	5

5. The facilitator(s) stimulated interest in the subject matter:

Not at All			Very Much	
1	2	3	4	5

6. The facilitator(s) encouraged group participation:

Not at All			Very Much	
1	2	3	4	5

7. Handouts or visual aids (if used) were:

Not Helpful		Very Helpful		
1	2	3	4	5

8. Any additional comments?

   ____

   ____

   ____

9. The most useful features of the session were:

   ____

   ____

   ____

10. Suggestions for improvement

    ____

    ____

    ____

11. Suggestions for topics related to this session

    ____

    ____

    ____

Communication: Session 2

FACILITATOR SELF-ASSESSMENT FORM

Directions: Please rate yourself from 1 to 5 on the following facilitator skills. The closer you are to a 5 within each domain, the more skilled you are at facilitation. We encourage you to complete this form prior to and after each teaching experience (e.g., a single session or an entire module). This will allow you to assess your performance as a facilitator over time.

Facilitator Behavior	1	2	3	4	5
Remains neutral					
Does not judge ideas					
Keeps the group focused on common task					
Asks clarifying questions					
Creates a climate free of criticism					
Encourages participation					
Structures participation					

Source: Adapted with permission from Welch, M. (1999). *Teaching diversity and cultural competence in health care: A trainer's guide.* San Francisco, CA: Perspectives of Differences Diversity Training and Consultation for Health Professionals (PODSDT).

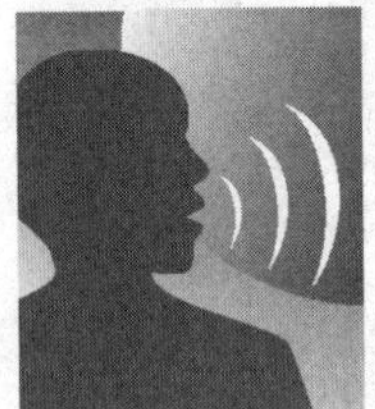

SESSION 2 (NONVIDEO OPTION):
Eliciting the Concerns of Children and Families

Session 2, Nonvideo Option, should be chosen if Nonvideo Option was used for Session 1.

At the beginning of the session, the facilitator and learners should introduce themselves briefly. (If the same group has recently completed Session 1, the facilitator may decide that introductions are not needed.) Ideas for creative introductions can be found in the Facilitator's Guide.

Setting the Context: The Bright Futures Concept

(May be omitted if recently presented or when sessions are combined.)

The facilitator **(F)** introduces the learners to the Bright Futures concept of health by reading or paraphrasing the following:

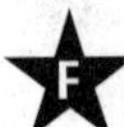 *The World Health Organization has defined health as "a state of complete physical, mental and social well-being and not merely the absence of disease or infirmity." Bright Futures embraces this broad definition of health—one that includes not only prevention of morbidity and mortality, but also the achievement of a child's full potential. In the Bright Futures concept of health, providing the capacity for healthy child development is as important as ameliorating illness or injury. Recognizing and acknowledging the strengths and resources of the child, family, and community are essential to promoting healthy growth and development.*

To build that capacity, the Pediatrics in Practice curriculum focuses on six core concepts: Partnership, Communication, Health Promotion/Illness Prevention, Time Management, Education, and Advocacy. The curriculum also includes a companion module (Health) and videotape that present an overview of Pediatrics in Practice and the Bright Futures approach.

Introducing the Session

Before introducing the session, the facilitator distributes the handout **Communication: Fostering Family-Centered Communication** to the learners. (The facilitator may choose not to distribute the handout if it was recently given to the same learners.)

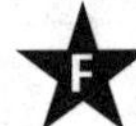 *Today's session is the second of three that comprise the* Pediatrics in Practice *Communication module.*

This session focuses on eliciting the needs and concerns of children and families. Family satisfaction with their health visit is intimately associated with the communication skills of the health professional. All too often, child health professionals do not elicit a family's important concerns. Children and their families leave their health visits with unmet needs. If a child or family feels that their concerns were not heard and addressed, the pediatric provider has lost the opportunity to provide comprehensive, quality health care and strengthen his or her relationship with the child and family.

Effective communication during health visits is essential to building trust and creating partnerships with children and families. Communication skills can be practiced and improved. Today we will use a reflective exercise to focus our attention on eliciting the concerns of children and families.

In today's session, our objectives will be to:

▶ *Focus on the communication skills required to elicit the needs and concerns of children and families*

▶ *Use a reflective exercise to focus our attention on communication styles and on identifying family concerns*

▶ *Compare provider-centered and patient- or family-centered communication styles*

When we have completed the session, you should be able to answer the following questions:

▶ How can I facilitate discussion during health visits with children and families?

▶ How do I determine the needs and concerns of children and families?

▶ What can I do to ensure that families leave the health visit with a feeling of confidence and a belief that their child's health care needs have been met?

Discussion and Exercises

Reflective Exercise

The facilitator describes the reflective exercise:

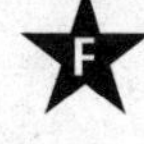 I would like each of you to spend 3 minutes considering the many health encounters that you have observed or experienced personally over the last year.

Slowly narrow your focus and concentrate on recreating one specific encounter in which the concerns of a child or family were not identified or met.

The facilitator distributes 3" x 5" index cards for those who find jotting a few notes helpful and allows 3 minutes for reflection without interruption.

After the 3 minutes of reflection, the facilitator initiates a "buzz group" discussion (people in small groups talking together around a particular focus), as follows:

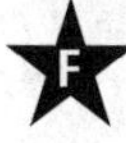 Now turn to the person sitting beside you and describe your experience as fully as possible in the next 2 minutes.

The facilitator writes these questions on a display board or flip chart and says:

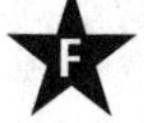 Try to address the following questions directly or indirectly as your story unfolds:

▶ In what context did this experience occur?

▶ What words, behaviors, questions, or mannerisms were used?

▶ What aspects of the encounter contributed to the family's concerns being missed and going unmet?

▶ Was the communication centered on the child and family or on the provider?

▶ What made the example so powerful and illustrative?

After the buzz group discussion period, the facilitator asks:

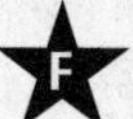 Who would like to describe their experience?

Discussion Questions and Answers

The facilitator continues the discussion and encourages all learners to offer their ideas and asks each of the following questions (one at a time).

 In your experience:

▶ What methods did the pediatric provider use to elicit the child or family's concerns?

▶ How successful was the provider in eliciting their concerns? Why or why not?

▶ What aspects of the health encounter contributed to the provider's failing to identify the concerns of the child or family?

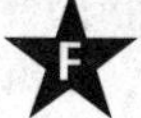 As you have observed, behaviors such as dominating the agenda, controlling the health interview, or using closed questions do not allow for discussion, negotiation, or partnership. These behaviors are usually associated with a provider-centered communication style.

If the encounter that you observed was provider centered:

▶ What are your impressions of this communication style?

▶ Was this style effective or ineffective in the encounter you experienced?

▶ What do you think about this communication style in general?

Provider-centered communication limits the effectiveness of the health interview by neglecting or ignoring the needs and concerns of the child and family.

The facilitator might continue with a discussion of communication styles in different circumstances.

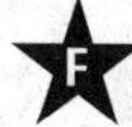 You might regard the provider-centered communication style as being typical of a surgeon, for instance, but we all vary our personal style to adapt to the circumstances of the moment. Provider-centered communication is not exclusive to surgeons. We com-

monly experience communication challenges due to time pressures, the settings in which we practice, or our own biases or perceptions about the seriousness of a family's concerns.

During residency training, you often find yourself in a variety of circumstances. You may be post-call or pre-call, or you may be in specific clinical settings such as the ER, continuity clinic, or an intensive care unit.

▶ Can you suggest some patient- or family-centered approaches to communication in these different circumstances?

▶ How would communication differ if patient- or family-centered methods (rather than provider-centered methods) were applied?

The facilitator refers to the **Communication: Fostering Family-Centered Communication** handout.

This handout highlights behaviors that help to determine a child or family's needs or concerns during a health encounter. Please take a moment to examine the list and identify specific behaviors that create a welcoming environment for open communication. You may want to reflect on asking open-ended questions and waiting for responses.

How much "wait time" do you provide in your encounters with children and families?

The facilitator continues:

Ideally, wait time should be at least 3 seconds following a question. This gives the child and family time to process the question. The wait may seem trivial, but if you actually observe health professionals in their encounters with families and look for evidence of the 3-second wait time, you will appreciate just how long 3 seconds can be. Wait time is essential in accomplishing the goal of eliciting the concerns of children and families.

Take-Home Message

The facilitator ends the session with the following:

The ability to elicit the needs and concerns of children and families is an essential communication skill in pediatric health care. In this session, we have examined some of your experiences in which families' needs went unmet. The discussion of those experiences helped to emphasize the effectiveness of patient- or family-centered communication and the disadvantages of provider-centered interactions. We have also explored the use of the 3-second wait time as a valuable tool in eliciting the true concerns of children and families. Before we conclude, what questions remain about what we addressed today?

Answers to the Guiding Questions

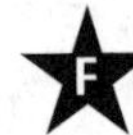

Now that we have completed this session on Communication, you should be able to answer the following questions:

▶ How can I facilitate discussion during health visits with children and families?

• Show interest and attention

• Appear patient and unhurried

• Use ordinary language, not medical jargon

• Encourage additional questions

▶ How do I determine the needs and concerns of children and families?

• Ask open-ended questions

• Wait at least 3 seconds for a response

• Ask follow-up questions

▶ What can I do to ensure that families leave the health visit with a feeling of confidence and a belief that their child's health care needs have been met?

• Encourage questions and answer them completely

• Give information clearly

• Draw pictures to clarify or demonstrate techniques

Planning for the Next Session (if Session 3 is planned)

The facilitator ends the session with the following:

In the next session, which focuses on evaluating communication skills, we will look at a variety of tools and forms that can assist you in assessing the effectiveness of your communication skills. As preparation for our next session, please think about some ways you

might receive feedback from the children and families you encounter in health visits.

(For those programs using a 2-hour workshop format, this could serve as a breakpoint and allow time for reflection.)

Evaluation

The facilitator now distributes the **Session Evaluation Form.** The facilitator also completes the **Facilitator Self-Assessment Form.**

Communication: Session 2

COMMUNICATION: FOSTERING FAMILY-CENTERED COMMUNICATION

Effective Behaviors

- Greet each family member and introduce self
- Use names of family members
- Incorporate social talk in the beginning of the interview
- Show interest and attention
- Demonstrate empathy
- Appear patient and unhurried
- Acknowledge concerns, fears, and feelings of child and family
- Use ordinary language, not medical jargon
- Use Bright Futures general and age-appropriate interview questions
- Give information clearly
- Query level of understanding and allow sufficient time for response
- Encourage additional questions
- Discuss family life, community, school

Active Listening Skills: Verbal Behaviors

- Allow child and parents to state concerns without interruption
- Encourage questions and answer them completely
- Clarify statements with follow-up questions
- Ask about feelings
- Acknowledge stress or difficulties
- Allow sufficient time for a response (wait time >3 seconds)
- Offer supportive comments
- Restate in the parent's or child's words
- Offer information or explanations

Active Listening Skills: Nonverbal Behaviors

- Nod in agreement
- Sit down at the level of the child and make eye contact
- Interact with or play with the child
- Show expression, attention, concern, or interest
- Convey understanding and empathy
- Touch child or parent (if appropriate)
- Draw pictures to clarify
- Demonstrate techniques

Source: Reproduced with permission from Green, M., Palfrey, J.S., Clark, E.M, & Anastasi, J.M. (Eds.) (2002). *Bright futures: Guidelines for health supervision of infants, children, and adolescents* (2nd ed., rev.)—*Pocket guide.* Arlington, VA: National Center for Education in Maternal and Child Health.

Communication: Session 2

SESSION EVALUATION FORM

Session 2: Eliciting the Concerns of Children and Families

Date: _______________________________

Facilitator(s): _______________________________

Site: _______________________________

1. Overall, I found the "Eliciting the Concerns of Children and Families" session to be:

Not Useful			Very Useful	
1	2	3	4	5

2. The objectives of the session were:

Not Clear				Clear
1	2	3	4	5

3. The organization of the session was:

Poor			Excellent	
1	2	3	4	5

4. The communication skills of the facilitator(s) were:

Poor			Excellent	
1	2	3	4	5

5. The facilitator(s) stimulated interest in the subject matter:

Not at All			Very Much	
1	2	3	4	5

6. The facilitator(s) encouraged group participation:

Not at All			Very Much	
1	2	3	4	5

7. Handouts or visual aids (if used) were:

Not Helpful		Very Helpful		
1	2	3	4	5

8. Any additional comments?

____
____
____

9. The most useful features of the session were:

____
____
____

10. Suggestions for improvement

____
____
____

11. Suggestions for topics related to this session

____
____
____

Communication: Session 2

FACILITATOR SELF-ASSESSMENT FORM

Directions: Please rate yourself from 1 to 5 on the following facilitator skills. The closer you are to a 5 within each domain, the more skilled you are at facilitation. We encourage you to complete this form prior to and after each teaching experience (e.g., a single session or an entire module). This will allow you to assess your performance as a facilitator over time.

Facilitator Behavior	1	2	3	4	5
Remains neutral					
Does not judge ideas					
Keeps the group focused on common task					
Asks clarifying questions					
Creates a climate free of criticism					
Encourages participation					
Structures participation					

Source: Adapted with permission from Welch, M. (1999). *Teaching diversity and cultural competence in health care: A trainer's guide.* San Francisco, CA: Perspectives of Differences Diversity Training and Consultation for Health Professionals (PODSDT).

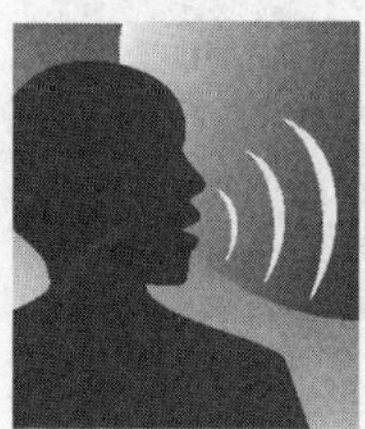

SESSION 3:
Individual and Group Assessment

At the beginning of the session, the facilitator and learners should introduce themselves briefly. (If the same group has recently completed Session 2, the facilitator may decide that introductions are not needed.) Ideas for creative introductions can be found in the Facilitator's Guide.

Setting the Context: The Bright Futures Concept

(May be omitted if recently presented or when sessions are combined.)

The facilitator **(F)** introduces the learners to the Bright Futures concept of health by reading or paraphrasing the following:

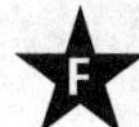 *The World Health Organization has defined health as "a state of complete physical, mental and social well-being and not merely the absence of disease or infirmity." Bright Futures embraces this broad definition of health—one that includes not only prevention of morbidity and mortality, but also the achievement of a child's full potential. In the Bright Futures concept of health, providing the capacity for healthy child development is as important as ameliorating illness or injury. Recognizing and acknowledging the strengths and resources of the child, family, and community are essential to promoting healthy growth and development.*

To build that capacity, the Pediatrics in Practice curriculum focuses on six core concepts: Partnership, Communication, Health Promotion/Illness Prevention, Time Management, Education, and Advocacy. The curriculum also includes a companion module (Health) and videotape that present an overview of Pediatrics in Practice and the Bright Futures approach.

Introducing the Session

Before introducing the session, the facilitator distributes the handout **Communication: Fostering Family-Centered Communication** to the learners. (The facilitator may choose not to distribute the handout if it was recently given to the same learners.)

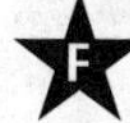 *Today's session is the last of three that comprise the* Pediatrics in Practice *Communication module.*

In our previous sessions, we have examined the need for effective communication among child health professionals and the children and families they serve. The importance of communication skills cannot be overemphasized. In medical practice, communication problems can contribute to family dissatisfaction, family noncompliance, medication errors, and even litigation.

Fortunately, communication is one area in which improvement is possible. Pediatric providers who assess their own performance or who receive evaluation from preceptors, families, or peers have the opportunity to refine their communication skills, provide comprehensive health care, and establish strong relationships with children and their families.

In today's session, our objective will be to:

▶ *Discuss a variety of communication skills, assessment tools, and forms*

When we have completed the session, you will have a variety of options for evaluating the effectiveness of your communication with the children and families you encounter each day.

Discussion and Exercises

There are several tools you can use to evaluate your communication skills in practice. Let's take a look at a few possible options for the evaluation of communication skills.

Individual Assessment

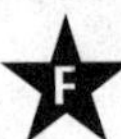
You may want to conduct an individual assessment that can be accomplished with the use of a self-reflective assessment form such as the one I am distributing to you now.

The facilitator distributes the **Learner Self-Assessment** handout and the **Preceptor Structured Observation Form** handout.

Take a moment to review the handout. This self-assessment form can be modified to meet your personal goals or to solicit specific evaluation from preceptors. You can decide how the form might be used for your own self-assessment and then for review with faculty preceptors.

You might want to request that your preceptors observe you directly with children and families during health visits. Then you can do a self-assessment and compare yours with the observations of your preceptor.

*For a more structured evaluation, I am also giving you the **Preceptor Structured Observation Form** (see page after the **Learner Self-Assessment**). This is an observation form for use by preceptors. You can review, discuss, and modify the checklist as needed.*

Group Assessment

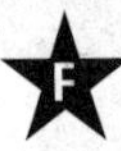
Another evaluation option you may want to use is group assessment. Please take a look at the patient and family survey form that I am distributing.

The facilitator gives the learners the **Patient and Family Survey Form.**

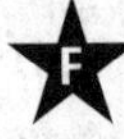
This form may also be modified for use in your various clinical environments. Let's discuss modifications that would be appropriate for the use of the form.

Optional Exercise

(Key individual faculty and learners should be recruited to take responsibility for this project.)

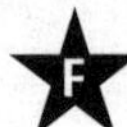
We are going to use this form as part of a communication skills evaluation project. As we examine the form and recommend modifications, we will include discussions of important methodological and logistical issues such as confidentiality, literacy, time, data collection, and data analysis.

A final session should be conducted to review the form modifications and the data obtained from either interviews or surveys.

Alternate Assessment Exercises

The facilitator and learners may choose to develop or explore additional methods of individual or group assessment. Some possibilities include:

1. Mock interviews with family actors (In some institutions, Parent Advisory Committees may be interested in supplying volunteers to act in this role and provide feedback about communication techniques.)
2. Videotaped interviews and reviews
3. Group or individual role-play
4. Peer observation and evaluation
5. Preceptor observation in continuity clinic or other practice settings using structured observation form

Some programs may want to conduct regular sessions in continuity clinic to review, reinforce, and highlight the importance of communication as a core Bright Futures concept.

Take-Home Message

The facilitator ends the session with the following:

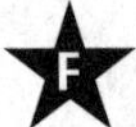
We know that communication skills are an essential aspect of family satisfaction and comprehensive health care. We also know that communication skills, such as active listening and effective patient- or family-centered communication behaviors, can be learned and improved.

In this session, we have discussed a variety of evaluation forms and exercises that you can use to improve your communication skills. I hope that you will continue to practice and refine your own skills in your encounters with children and families each day. Before we conclude, what questions remain about what we addressed today?

The facilitator may want to discuss the learners' interest in an optional fourth session, 3 to 4 weeks later, to assess the impact of the Communication module after learners have had the opportunity to practice skills and obtain feedback from patients, families, and faculty.

New clinic projects may evolve around related communication issues such as personality style, interpersonal dynamics, and multicultural issues, including the use of interpreters.

Evaluation

The facilitator now distributes the **Session Evaluation Form** and the **Module Evaluation Form.** The facilitator also completes the **Facilitator Self-Assessment Form.**

Communication: Session 3

COMMUNICATION: FOSTERING FAMILY-CENTERED COMMUNICATION

Effective Behaviors

- Greet each family member and introduce self
- Use names of family members
- Incorporate social talk in the beginning of the interview
- Show interest and attention
- Demonstrate empathy
- Appear patient and unhurried
- Acknowledge concerns, fears, and feelings of child and family
- Use ordinary language, not medical jargon
- Use Bright Futures general and age-appropriate interview questions
- Give information clearly
- Query level of understanding and allow sufficient time for response
- Encourage additional questions
- Discuss family life, community, school

Active Listening Skills: Verbal Behaviors

- Allow child and parents to state concerns without interruption
- Encourage questions and answer them completely
- Clarify statements with follow-up questions
- Ask about feelings
- Acknowledge stress or difficulties
- Allow sufficient time for a response (wait time >3 seconds)
- Offer supportive comments
- Restate in the parent's or child's words
- Offer information or explanations

Active Listening Skills: Nonverbal Behaviors

- Nod in agreement
- Sit down at the level of the child and make eye contact
- Interact with or play with the child
- Show expression, attention, concern, or interest
- Convey understanding and empathy
- Touch child or parent (if appropriate)
- Draw pictures to clarify
- Demonstrate techniques

Source: Reproduced with permission from Green, M., Palfrey, J.S., Clark, E.M, & Anastasi, J.M. (Eds.) (2002). *Bright futures: Guidelines for health supervision of infants, children, and adolescents* (2nd ed., rev.)—*Pocket guide.* Arlington, VA: National Center for Education in Maternal and Child Health.

Communication: Session 3

LEARNER SELF-ASSESSMENT FORM

SELF-ASSESSMENT OF COMMUNICATION SKILLS					
Communication Skill	**Undeveloped <—> Developing <—> Mastered**				
Ability to establish a close relationship with children	1	2	3	4	5
Ability to establish a close relationship with families	1	2	3	4	5
Skill in identifying the needs and concerns of children	1	2	3	4	5
Skill in identifying the needs and concerns of families	1	2	3	4	5
Use of active listening in my interviews with children	1	2	3	4	5
Use of active listening in my interviews with families	1	2	3	4	5
Adaptability of communication style	1	2	3	4	5
Overall impression of skills in interviewing and communication	1	2	3	4	5

Communication: Session 3

PRECEPTOR STRUCTURED OBSERVATION FORM

EFFECTIVE BEHAVIORS IN PATIENT- OR FAMILY-CENTERED COMMUNICATION		
	Observed with:	
Behavior	*Child*	*Family*
Uses names of family members and children		
Incorporates social talk in the beginning of the visit		
Shows interest and attention		
Demonstrates empathy		
Appears patient and unhurried		
Acknowledges concerns, fears, and feelings of the patient and family		
Allows family members to state concerns without interrupting		
When age appropriate, allows child to state concerns		
Uses ordinary language, not medical jargon		
Uses age-appropriate Interview Questions from *Bright Futures Pocket Guide*		
Gives information clearly		
Queries level of understanding and uses wait time (>3 seconds)		
Encourages additional questions		
Discusses family, community, and school		

Communication: Session 3

PATIENT AND FAMILY SURVEY FORM

To our Patients and Families:

The child health professionals in our clinic are very interested in your opinions about the care that we provide for you and your child. As part of our effort to continue to improve the care we offer, we ask that you please complete this survey about today's visit. Your responses will be confidential and will not be shared directly with your child health professional.

Thank you for your time in completing this survey.

The Staff of the Clinic

PATIENT AND FAMILY SURVEY	I am a: ☐ Patient ☐ Family Member				
My Child Health Professional:	**Disagree <—> Uncertain <—> Agree**				
Answered the concerns I had about my child	1	2	3	4	5
Listened to me and my child and respected our feelings	1	2	3	4	5
Included me in decisions	1	2	3	4	5
Presented information clearly so that I could understand	1	2	3	4	5
Helped me feel confident and reassured	1	2	3	4	5
Paid attention to me and my concerns	1	2	3	4	5
Gave me enough time to talk about my concerns	1	2	3	4	5
Provided me and my child with very good care	1	2	3	4	5

Comments

____

____

____

____

____

____

Communication: Session 3

SESSION EVALUATION FORM

Session 3: Individual and Group Assessment

Date: _______________________________

Facilitator(s): _______________________________

Site: _______________________________

---

1. Overall, I found the "Individual and Group Assessment" session to be:

Not Useful			Very Useful	
1	2	3	4	5

2. The objectives of the session were:

Not Clear				Clear
1	2	3	4	5

3. The organization of the session was:

Poor				Excellent
1	2	3	4	5

4. The communication skills of the facilitator(s) were:

Poor				Excellent
1	2	3	4	5

5. The facilitator(s) stimulated interest in the subject matter:

Not at All			Very Much	
1	2	3	4	5

6. The facilitator(s) encouraged group participation:

Not at All			Very Much	
1	2	3	4	5

7. Handouts or visual aids (if used) were:

Not Helpful		Very Helpful		
1	2	3	4	5

8. Any additional comments?

____

____

____

9. The most useful features of the session were:

____

____

____

10. Suggestions for improvement

____

____

____

11. Suggestions for topics related to this session

____

____

____

Communication: Session 3

MODULE EVALUATION FORM

Please indicate the effectiveness of this module in developing an awareness and under-standing of the use of communication skills in child health visits.

Sessions on:	Not effective <—> Highly effective				
1. Learning to listen actively	1	2	3	4	5
2. Eliciting the concerns of children and families	1	2	3	4	5
3. Individual and group assessment	1	2	3	4	5
4. Discussions and exercises in general	1	2	3	4	5

Comments

____

____

____

____

____

____

____

____

Communication: Session 3

FACILITATOR SELF-ASSESSMENT FORM

Directions: Please rate yourself from 1 to 5 on the following facilitator skills. The closer you are to a 5 within each domain, the more skilled you are at facilitation. We encourage you to complete this form prior to and after each teaching experience (e.g., a single session or an entire module). This will allow you to assess your performance as a facilitator over time.

Facilitator Behavior	1	2	3	4	5
Remains neutral					
Does not judge ideas					
Keeps the group focused on common task					
Asks clarifying questions					
Creates a climate free of criticism					
Encourages participation					
Structures participation					

Source: Adapted with permission from Welch, M. (1999). *Teaching diversity andcultural competence in health care: A trainer's guide.* San Francisco, CA: Perspectives of Differences Diversity Training and Consultation for Health Professionals (PODSDT).

References

Benjamin, J.T., Cimino, S.A., & Hafler, J.P., Bright Futures Health Promotion Work Group, & Bernstein, H.H. (2002). The office visit: A time to promote health—but how? *Contemporary Pediatrics, 19*(2), 90–107.

Ferris, T.G., Saglam, D., Satfford, R.S., Causino, N., Starfield, B., Culpepper, L., & Blumenthal, D. (1998). Changes in the daily practice of primary care for children. *Archives of Pediatrics and Adolescent Medicine, 152,* 227.

Green, M., & Palfrey, J.S. (Eds.) (2002). *Bright futures: Guidelines for gealth supervision of infants, children, and adolescents* (2nd ed., rev.). Arlington, VA: National Center for Education in Maternal and Child Health.

Green, M., Palfrey, J.S., Clark, E.M., & Anastasi, J.M. (Eds.) (2002). *Bright futures: Guidelines for health supervision of infants, children, and adolescents* (2nd ed., rev.)—*Pocket guide.* Arlington, VA: National Center for Education in Maternal and Child Health.

Haines, R. [dir.] (1991). *The doctor* [film]. Burbank, CA: Touchstone Pictures, Silver Screen Partners IV.

Morgan, E.R., & Winter, R.J. (1996). Teaching communication skills: An essential part of residency training. *Archives of Pediatrics and Adolescent Medicine, 150,* 638.

Ong, L.M.L., deHaes. J.C.J.M., Hoos, A.M., & Lammes, F.B. (1995). Doctor-patient communication: A review of the literature. *Social Science Medicine, 40*(7), 903.

Palfrey, J.S. (1998). Comprehensive child health: Is it in the picture? *Archives of Pediatrics and Adolescent Medicine, 152,* 222.

Rogers, C.R., & Farson, R.E. (1975). *Active listening* (new ed.). Chicago: University of Chicago, Industrial Relations Center.

Werner, E.R., Adler, R., Robinson, R., & Korsch, B.M. (1979). Attitudes and interpersonal skills during pediatric internship. *Pediatrics, 63,* 491.

Young, K.T., Davis, K., Schoen, C., & Parker, S. (1998). Listening to parents: A national survey of parents with young children. *Archives of Pediatrics and Adolescent Medicine, 152,* 255.

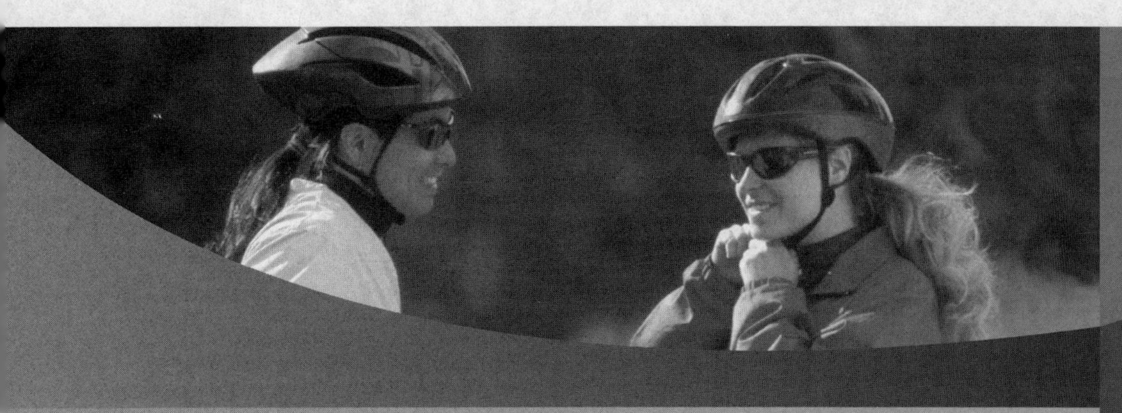

Chapter 5

Health Promotion

Promoting Health and Preventing Illness

John T. Benjamin
Habib Shariat
Judith S. Shaw

CONTENTS

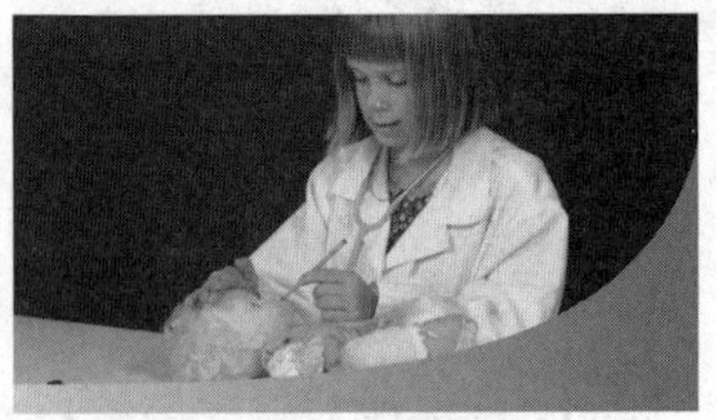

HEALTH PROMOTION
Promoting Health and Preventing Illness

OVERVIEW

Background

Child health professionals are in a unique position to promote health and prevent illness. They have frequent interactions with children and families, particularly in the early years. These encounters give child health professionals ample opportunities to observe, listen to, and recognize issues in promoting health and preventing illness. Because families often hesitate to initiate discussions on these topics, it is essential that child health professionals identify and focus on the needs and concerns of each child and family. Determining relevant health promotion topics; personalizing guidance; making use of family and community resources; and achieving partnership and understanding with the family are all fundamental components of effective health promotion and illness prevention.

Goal

The overall goal of this module is to encourage openness between the child health professional, child, and family by emphasizing the importance of tailoring health care to fit the individual and of recognizing pertinent health promotion and illness prevention issues.

This module will enable learners to:

▶ Ask effective interview and follow-up questions

▶ Determine relevant health promotion and illness prevention topics

▶ Provide personalized guidance

▶ Use family and community resources

▶ Identify and overcome barriers to optimal health care

Instructional Design

This module consists of three 30-minute sessions.

▶ Session 1 introduces the effective use of interview and follow-up questions and presents useful approaches to providing personalized guidance.

▶ Session 2 reinforces the use of effective questions and focuses on the identification and use of family and community resources.

▶ Each of the two sessions can be used as a separate, stand-alone offering, or the sessions can be combined. See the Facilitator's Guide for information on combining sessions.

▶ Session 3 is optional and elaborates on the information taught in the previous two sessions.

Teaching Strategies

The teaching strategies used in this module include case discussion, reflective exercise, and brainstorming. These strategies have been selected to help learners develop the skills required to convey meaningful health-promoting messages and strategies for each health care encounter with children and their families. Please refer to the Facilitator's Guide for more information related to each strategy.

Evaluation

Learners will complete a Session Evaluation Form following each session. Facilitators are encouraged to complete a Facilitator Self-Assessment Form prior to and following each teaching experience (e.g., a single session or an entire module) in order to assess their performance over time.

In addition, three optional evaluation forms—a **Preceptor Structured Observation Form**, a **Learner Self-Assessment Form**, and a **Patient and Family Survey Form**—are included at the end of each session. These forms can be used following each session and/or following the completion of the entire module.

Guiding Questions

Learners who have completed the entire Health Promotion module should be able to answer the following questions:

▶ How can I effectively identify relevant health promotion and illness prevention topics?

▶ How can I ensure that I give personalized guidance?

▶ How can I identify and use family and community resources to promote health and prevent illness?

INTRODUCTION TO TEACHING SESSIONS

Session 1: Identifying Relevant Health Promotion Topics

Objectives

The objectives for this session are for the facilitator to:

▶ Introduce the effective use of interview and follow-up questions in determining the health promotion topics important to each family

▶ Present useful approaches to providing personalized guidance, directing families to community resources, and achieving understanding with the family

Materials

The materials and teaching aids needed for this session are:

Handouts

▶ Health Promotion: Promoting Health and Preventing Illness

▶ Case Vignette: Manuel's Anemia Referral

▶ Age-Specific Interview and Follow-up Questions

▶ Session Evaluation Form

▶ Preceptor Structured Observation Form (optional)

▶ Learner Self-Assessment Form (optional)

▶ Patient and Family Survey Form (optional)

Facilitator Form

▶ Facilitator Self-Assessment Form

Teaching Aids

▶ Display board, flip chart, or chalkboard

▶ Markers or chalk

Time

The time allocated for this session is 30 minutes.

Session 2: Asking Questions and Identifying Resources

Objectives

The objectives for this session are for the facilitator to:

▶ Review the importance of asking open-ended interview questions and recognizing verbal and nonverbal cues

▶ Encourage the use of family and community resources in promoting health and preventing illness

Materials

The materials and teaching aids needed for this session are:

Handouts

▶ Health Promotion: Promoting Health and Preventing Illness

▶ Case Vignette: Antoine's 2 Week Visit

▶ Session Evaluation Form

▶ Preceptor Structured Observation Form (optional)

▶ Learner Self-Assessment Form (optional)

▶ Patient and Family Survey Form (optional)

Facilitator Form

▶ Facilitator Self-Assessment Form

Teaching Aids

▶ Display board, flip chart, or chalkboard
▶ Markers or chalk

Time

The time allocated for this session is 30 minutes.

Session 3 (Optional): A Reflective Exercise

Objectives

The objectives for this session are for the facilitator to:

▶ Encourage learners to relate their own experiences with health promotion and illness prevention
▶ Give learners the opportunity to apply their skills in asking interview and follow-up questions, giving personalized guidance, and incorporating family and community resources to their cases
▶ Invite learners to share effective methods for overcoming health care barriers

Materials

The materials and teaching aids needed for this session are:

Handouts

▶ Health Promotion: Promoting Health and Preventing Illness
▶ Reflective Exercise
▶ Alternate Case Vignettes (if reflective exercise is not chosen)
▶ Session Evaluation Form
▶ Preceptor Structured Observation Form (optional)
▶ Learner Self-Assessment Form (optional)
▶ Patient and Family Survey Form (optional)

Facilitator Form

▶ Facilitator Self-Assessment Form

Teaching Aids

▶ Display board, flip chart, or chalkboard
▶ Markers or chalk

Time

The time allocated for this session is 30 minutes.

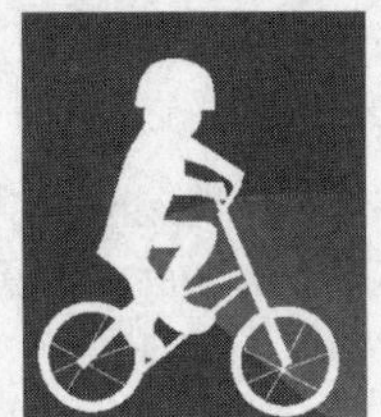

SESSION 1:
Identifying Relevant Health Promotion Topics

At the beginning of the session, the facilitator and learners should introduce themselves briefly. Ideas for creative introductions can be found in the Facilitator's Guide.

Setting the Context: The Bright Futures Concept

The facilitator **(F)** introduces the learners to the Bright Futures concept of health by reading or paraphrasing the following:

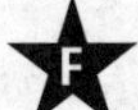 *The World Health Organization has defined health as "a state of complete physical, mental and social well-being and not merely the absence of disease or infirmity." Bright Futures embraces this broad definition of health—one that includes not only prevention of morbidity and mortality, but also the achievement of a child's full potential. In the Bright Futures concept of health, providing the capacity for healthy child development is as important as ameliorating illness or injury. Recognizing and acknowledging the strengths and resources of the child, family, and community are essential to promoting healthy growth and development.*

To build that capacity, the Pediatrics in Practice *curriculum focuses on six core concepts: Partnership, Communication, Health Promotion/Illness Prevention, Time Management, Education, and Advocacy. The curriculum also includes a companion module (Health) and videotape that present an overview of* Pediatrics in Practice *and the Bright Futures approach.*

Introducing the Session

Before introducing the session, the facilitator distributes the handout **Health Promotion: Promoting Health and Preventing Illness** to the learners.

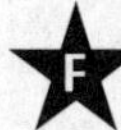 *Today's session is the first of three that comprise the* Pediatrics in Practice *Health Promotion module.*

As child health professionals, you are in a unique position to promote health and prevent illness. You have frequent interactions with children and families, particularly in the early years. These encounters give you ample opportunities to observe, listen to, and recognize issues in promoting health and preventing illness. Families may have questions about the seriousness of an illness; concerns about expenses; anxiety about child care issues; family issues such as divorce or separation; work-related issues; or even concerns about their own fitness as parents. Because families often hesitate to initiate discussions on these topics with child health professionals, it is essential that you identify and focus on the needs and concerns of each child and family.

In today's session, our objectives will be to:

▶ *Focus on the importance of asking open-ended interview and directed follow-up questions in order to elicit a family's concerns during a health visit*

▶ *Examine a specific case to demonstrate the use of interview and follow-up questions to promote health and prevent illness.*

When we have completed the session, you should be able to answer the following questions:

▶ *How can I effectively identify relevant health promotion and illness prevention topics?*

▶ *How can I ensure that I give personalized guidance?*

The facilitator distributes copies of the case vignette handout **Manuel's Anemia Referral** to learners and either reads the case aloud or asks one of the learners to do so.

 *This case about Manuel will demonstrate how asking open-ended questions, followed by asking focused questions, can help to identify problems specific to each child.*

Discussion and Exercises

Use of Interview Questions

Ask Open-ended Interview Questions

The facilitator asks the learners one or more of the following questions:

- *What are your impressions and reactions to this case?*
- *What might you want to address and explore further?*
- *What questions would you ask and how would you ask them?*

The facilitator records the learners' answers on a display board. Some responses might include:

- Adequacy of diet
- Past medical history
- Family and social history

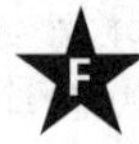 *What are some nonjudgmental interview questions you would want to ask the mother?*

The facilitator again records the learners' responses as they brainstorm about possible questions to ask Manuel's mother.

If the learners are not responding, the following are examples of appropriate interview questions that might be used to stimulate discussion:

About diet:
- Please tell me what Manuel usually eats each day. What kinds of food does he like?

About past medical history:
- Please tell me about your pregnancy, labor, and delivery.
- What concerns do you have about Manuel's health now? Have you had any in the past?
- What aspects of his behavior worry you?

About social and family history:
- Who lives with you and Manuel in your home?
- Tell me about where you are living now.

After the questions are listed on the display board, the facilitator asks the learners:

 *Which questions do you think were the most effective interview questions? Which were less effective?*

The facilitator summarizes by noting:

- *Effective questions are open ended and nonjudgmental.*
- *Good questions allow the child health professional to ask follow-up questions.*
- *Ineffective questions are those that invite yes or no answers and may imply judgment of behaviors.*

The facilitator continues the session, telling the learners that the open-ended questions revealed the following information:

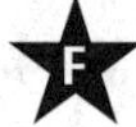
- *Beatrice's husband left her 6 months ago.*
- *Beatrice and Manuel moved in with Beatrice's sister and her children.*
- *The living conditions in the apartment are not good. There is often no heat, and the paint is peeling.*
- *Beatrice is quite concerned about the effects of this situation on Manuel.*

Ask Directed Follow-up Questions

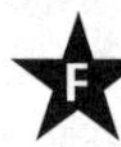 *Your initial questions have disclosed the family's concerns. The next step is to ask directed follow-up questions that will elicit more information from the family.*

Examples:

About diet:
- What does Manuel eat for breakfast? For lunch? And for dinner?
- Children seem to put everything in their mouths. Have you ever seen Manuel or his cousins eat any of the peeling paint in the apartment?

About medical history:
- You've already told me about your pregnancy with Manuel. Was he delivered on time or was he born early? How much did he weigh?
- Do you think he's growing like other children his age, or do you think there's a difference?
- Has Manuel ever been tested for anemia or lead poisoning? If so, do you remember the results?

About social and family history:

▶ What changes have moving in with your sister brought for you and Manuel?

▶ Is Manuel's father involved in his care at all?

▶ Have your sister's children ever had problems with anemia or lead poisoning?

The facilitator tells the learners that the directed follow-up questions have provided the following additional information:

▶ *Beatrice has noticed that Manuel and her sister's children have eaten some of the paint chips.*

▶ *Beatrice has been concerned about Manuel's development.*

▶ *Manuel has never been anemic or had lead poisoning.*

▶ *Beatrice must support herself since Manuel's father is no longer in the picture.*

The facilitator also reveals:

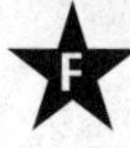

When Manuel's lab results return the next day, they show that his hemoglobin is low at 10.8 gms%, and his venous lead level is quite elevated at 45 mcg/dl.

In this example, we see that the initial open-ended interview questions, combined with the more specific, directed follow-up questions, uncovered the needed diagnosis of lead poisoning.

Using the display board, the facilitator creates the following chart to compare the two types of questions and to clarify the major differences.

Interview Questions	Directed Follow-up Questions
• Are open ended	• Focus the discussion
• Are nonjudgmental	• Seek specific information
• Allow for follow-up questions	• Can be answered with yes or no

Working with the Family

Give Personalized Guidance

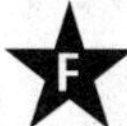

When the family returns to get Manuel's laboratory results, you will want to help them understand the information and to provide personalized guidance.

How would you share this information with the family?

Some examples might include:

▶ Explain the results of the WIC evaluation and the laboratory results.

▶ Explain that when a child has an elevated blood lead level, the Department of Health is contacted to assist in checking the home. Explain that the family should be helped in finding other housing while the lead is being removed.

▶ Advise Beatrice that Manuel's cousins should be tested for lead poisoning.

▶ Discuss the need to temporarily remove Manuel and his family from the apartment if peeling paint or another source of lead is found.

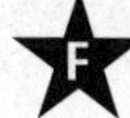

While it's important that you explain the medical aspects of the case (such as interventions), you also want to involve the family in the discussion about how to deal with the problem.

Incorporate Family and Community Resources

The facilitator asks the learners to suggest various resources that could be used in this case. To help focus the discussion, the facilitator writes on the display board the following words: "Child/Family—Community."

Listed below are some possibilities that the learners might suggest for each category:

Child and family:

▶ Arrange to have the amount of lead in the apartment analyzed.

▶ If the apartment shows a large amount of lead, discuss options available to Beatrice and her sister (either remove the source of the lead or move out of the apartment).

▶ Discuss the problem with the family's landlord and with the local health department.

Community:

▶ Work with the local health department to identify other children in the building who might have been exposed.

▶ Work with the health department to identify areas of high lead and try to get the problem corrected.

 Serve as a referral site for testing other children.

Come to Closure with the Family

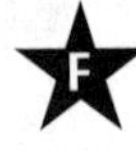 *At the end of the visit, you want to be sure that the family understands what is being done and what has been decided.*

What would be a good way to end the health visit?

Possible examples might include the following:

▶ What questions do you have about what we discussed today?

▶ What other concerns do you have about your child's health?

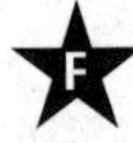 *Answers to these questions might identify barriers to the guidance you have given and the care you have prescribed.*

Examples of such barriers include:

▶ Lack of transportation

▶ Poor relationship with the landlord

▶ Limited financial assistance to find alternative housing

Take-Home Message

The facilitator ends the session with the following:

 *The case vignette in this session demonstrates the importance of good interview questions, careful listening, and specific follow-up questions in identifying relevant health promotion topics.*

Without the right interview questions, a child health professional might not have been aware that Beatrice had recently moved in with her sister and that Manuel was at risk for lead poisoning. This case also illustrates techniques that you, as a child health professional, can use to involve the family and community in handling a health promotion or illness prevention issue. Before we conclude, what questions remain about what we addressed today?

The facilitator then distributes the **Age-Specific Interview and Follow-up Questions** handout and says:

This handout illustrates sample interview and follow-up questions (adaptable for use with parents). Please review the handout, and if you have any questions, we can answer them during clinic today or at another time.

Answers to the Guiding Questions

 *Now that we have completed this session on Health Promotion, you should be able to answer the following questions:*

▶ How can I effectively identify relevant health promotion and illness prevention topics?

● Ask effective open-ended and nonjudgmental interview questions to obtain information

● Ask directed follow-up questions to focus the discussion and communicate understanding

● Listen to and recognize nonverbal cues during encounters with patients and families

▶ How can I ensure that I give personalized guidance?

● Introduce new information and reinforce healthy practices based on responses to your questions and facts obtained in the medical, social, and family history

● Identify and address any barriers to care

The facilitator explains:

 *The child health professional, the family, or the community might present a barrier to optimal health care. The following are some examples:*

The child health professional may:

▶ Encounter lack of trust by the family

▶ Lack confidence in the role of child health professional

▶ Experience scheduling difficulties

▶ Lack adequate time with patients

The family may:

▶ Be afraid or anxious

▶ Lack information or be in denial

▶ Have inadequate resources

▶ Experience spousal, grandparent, or sibling problems

The community may:

▶ Not have pediatric and family-centered hospitals

▶ Lack responsive social services

Planning for the Next Session (if Session 2 is planned)

 *In our next session, we will look at another case and review the importance of asking open-ended and follow-up questions. We will also discuss the use of family and community resources. As you prepare for the next session, please consider the following question:*

> ▶ *How can I identify and use family and community resources to promote health and prevent illness?*

Evaluation

The facilitator now distributes the **Session Evaluation Form**. The facilitator also completes the **Facilitator Self-Assessment Form.**

Health Promotion: Session 1

HEALTH PROMOTION: PROMOTING HEALTH AND PREVENTING ILLNESS

It is essential that health professionals identify and focus on the individual needs and concerns of the child and family, since families often hesitate to initiate discussion.

1. Identify relevant health promotion topics.

- Ask open-ended, nonjudgmental questions to obtain information and identify appropriate guidance
  Example:
  - *"How is breastfeeding going? What questions/concerns do you have today?"*
- Ask specific follow-up questions to communicate understanding and focus the discussion
  Example:
  - *"How often and for how long do you breastfeed Manuel? How do you tell when he wants to be fed?"*
- Listen for verbal and nonverbal cues to discover underlying or unidentified concerns
  Example:
  - *"How do you balance your roles of partner and parent? When do you make time for yourself?"*
  Note:
  - *If parent hesitates with an answer, try to determine the reason.*
  - *If parent brings in child multiple times for minor problems, explore the possibility of another unresolved concern.*

2. Give personalized guidance.

- Introduce new information and reinforce healthy practices
  Examples:
  - *Take time for self, time with partner*
  - *Encourage partner to help care for baby*
  - *Accept support from friends, family*

3. Incorporate family and community resources.

- Approach child within context of family and community
- Identify each family member's role
  Examples:
  - *"Who helps you with Kim?"*
  - *"How much rest are you getting?"*
- Identify community resources such as lactation consultant or local La Leche League chapter
- Develop working relationships with community professionals, and establish lines of referral
- Create a list of local resources with contact information

4. Come to closure.

- Be sure that the health message is understood
  Examples:
  - *"Have I addressed your concerns?"*
  - *"Do you have any other concerns about Kim's health?"*
- Identify possible barriers
  Example:
  - *"What problems do you think you might have following through with what we discussed today?"*

Source: Reproduced with permission from Green. M., Palfrey, J.S., Clark, E.M., & Anastasi, J.M. (Eds.) (2002). *Bright futures: Guidelines for health supervision of infants, children, and adolescents* (2nd ed., rev.)—*Pocket guide.* Arlington, VA: National Center for Education in Maternal and Child Health.

Health Promotion: Session 1

CASE VIGNETTE: MANUEL'S ANEMIA REFERRAL

Manuel is a 2-year-old child who has been referred to you by his local health department because of a low hemoglobin found on routine screening for WIC. He has had no hospitalizations and has had routine check-ups and all immunizations performed at the health department.

When you enter the examining room, Manuel is noisily running around the room and tries to get into the trash can. His mother, Beatrice, gently diverts him by reading him a story.

Manuel's physical examination is normal. His height and weight are at the 25th percentile, and his development seems appropriate for his age.

Health Promotion: Session 1

AGE-SPECIFIC INTERVIEW AND FOLLOW-UP QUESTIONS

Adaptable for use with parents

Interview Questions (open-ended)	Follow-up Questions (directed)
Age of Child: 8 years old	
How is school going?	What grade are you in? What grades do you get?
Tell me about your friends.	What are their names?
What do you like to do together?	How often do you [take part in that activity]?
What are the rules at home regarding food, movies, games, or safety?	Do you follow these rules?
What are some things you are good at?	Can you describe them?
What feedback do you get from your teacher about your school performance?	Do you have trouble getting your work done on time?
What do you do for fun?	What after-school activities do you do? What do you like to read?
Are there any issues that you are concerned about?	Can you describe them? What specifically concerns you?
How do you make sure that you are safe when you bike or play sports?	Do you wear a helmet? Do you know how to swim?
Age of Child: 15 years old	
How are you doing in school?	What grade are you in? What grades do you get?
Tell me about some things you are really good at.	Can you describe them?
What makes you sad, angry, or worried?	Do you talk about these things to anyone? Who do you talk to?
What do you do when you feel down or depressed? Have you ever thought about harming yourself?	Is there anyone you talk to about these feelings?
Is there anything you would like to change about the way you look?	If yes, do you diet or exercise excessively? Do you purge?
Tell me about others you know who use alcohol or drugs.	Do you drink? How much do you drink? What drugs have you tried?
Tell me about your social life.	Do you date? One person or more than one? Are you sexually active?

Health Promotion: Session 1

SESSION EVALUATION FORM

Session 1: Identifying Relevant Health Promotion Topics

Date: ___________________________

Facilitator(s): ___________________________

Site: ___________________________

---

1. Overall, I found the "Identifying Relevant Health Promotion Topics" session to be:

Not Useful				Very Useful
1	2	3	4	5

2. The objectives of the session were:

Not Clear				Clear
1	2	3	4	5

3. The organization of the session was:

Poor				Excellent
1	2	3	4	5

4. The communication skills of the facilitator(s) were:

Poor				Excellent
1	2	3	4	5

5. The facilitator(s) stimulated interest in the subject matter:

Not at All				Very Much
1	2	3	4	5

6. The facilitator(s) encouraged group participation:

Not at All				Very Much
1	2	3	4	5

7. Handouts or visual aids (if used) were:

Not Helpful				Very Helpful
1	2	3	4	5

8. Any additional comments?

   ____

   ____

   ____

9. The most useful features of the session were:

   ____

   ____

   ____

10. Suggestions for improvement

    ____

    ____

    ____

11. Suggestions for topics related to this session

    ____

    ____

    ____

Health Promotion: Session 1

FACILITATOR SELF-ASSESSMENT FORM

Directions: Please rate yourself from 1 to 5 on the following facilitator skills. The closer you are to a 5 within each domain, the more skilled you are at facilitation. We encourage you to complete this form prior to and after each teaching experience (e.g., a single session or an entire module). This will allow you to assess your performance as a facilitator over time.

Facilitator Behavior	1	2	3	4	5
Remains neutral					
Does not judge ideas					
Keeps the group focused on common task					
Asks clarifying questions					
Creates a climate free of criticism					
Encourages participation					
Structures participation					

Source: Adapted with permission from Welch, M. (1999). *Teaching diversity and cultural competence in health care: A trainer's guide.* San Francisco, CA: Perspectives of Differences Diversity Training and Consultation for Health Professionals (PODSDT).

Health Promotion: Session 1

PRECEPTOR STRUCTURED OBSERVATION FORM

Behavior	Observed	Not Observed	Not Applicable
Asked open-ended questions to obtain information			
Followed up with more specific questions			
Communicated understanding to the child and/or family			
Gave personalized guidance and introduced new information			
Identified each family member's role in the care of the child			
Identified community resources if applicable			
Came to closure by making sure that the health message was understood			
Identified and addressed any health care barriers			

Health Promotion: Session 1

LEARNER SELF-ASSESSMENT FORM

During health visits today, I feel that I:	Circle: 1 = disagree to 5 = agree				
Asked open-ended questions to obtain information	1	2	3	4	5
Followed up with more specific questions	1	2	3	4	5
Communicated understanding to the child and/or family	1	2	3	4	5
Gave personalized guidance and introduced new information	1	2	3	4	5
Identified each family member's role in the care of the child	1	2	3	4	5
Identified community resources if applicable	1	2	3	4	5
Came to closure by making sure that the health message was understood	1	2	3	4	5
Identified and addressed any health care barriers	1	2	3	4	5

Health Promotion: Session 1

PATIENT AND FAMILY SURVEY FORM

To our Patients and Families:

The child health professionals in our clinic are very interested in your opinions about the care that we provide for you and your child. As part of our effort to continue to improve the care we offer, we ask that you please complete this survey about today's visit. Your responses will be confidential and will not be shared directly with your child health professional.

Thank you for your time in completing this survey.

The Staff of the Clinic

FAMILY SURVEY	Respondent is: ☐ Child ☐ Family				
My Child Health Professional:	**Disagree**	**<—>**	**Uncertain**	**<—>**	**Agree**
Addressed the concerns I had about my child	1	2	3	4	5
Listened to me and my child and respected our feelings	1	2	3	4	5
Involved me in decisions	1	2	3	4	5
Talked so that I could understand	1	2	3	4	5
Helped me feel better about my child	1	2	3	4	5
Seemed to care about me and my child	1	2	3	4	5
Gave me adequate time to discuss my concerns	1	2	3	4	5
Provided high-quality care	1	2	3	4	5

Comments

____

____

____

____

____

____

____

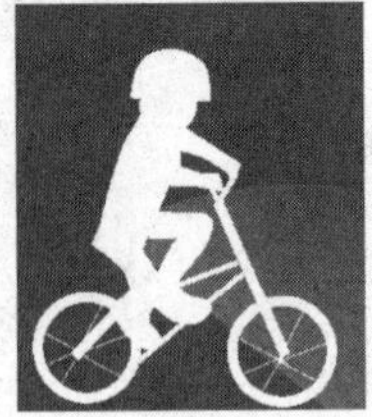

SESSION 2:
Asking Questions and Identifying Resources

At the beginning of the session, the facilitator and learners should introduce themselves briefly. (If the same group has recently completed Session 1, the facilitator may decide that introductions are not needed.) Ideas for creative introductions can be found in the Facilitator's Guide.

Setting the Context: The Bright Futures Concept

(May be omitted if recently presented or when sessions are combined.)

The facilitator **(F)** introduces the learners to the Bright Futures concept of health by reading or paraphrasing the following:

 *The World Health Organization has defined health as "a state of complete physical, mental and social well-being and not merely the absence of disease or infirmity." Bright Futures embraces this broad definition of health—one that includes not only prevention of morbidity and mortality, but also the achievement of a child's full potential. In the Bright Futures concept of health, providing the capacity for healthy child development is as important as ameliorating illness or injury. Recognizing and acknowledging the strengths and resources of the child, family, and community are essential to promoting healthy growth and development.*

To build that capacity, this Pediatrics in Practice curriculum focuses on six core concepts: Partnership, Communication, Health Promotion/Illness Prevention, Time Management, Education, and Advocacy. The curriculum also includes a companion module (Health) and videotape that present an overview of Pediatrics in Practice and the Bright Futures approach.

Introducing the Session

Before introducing the session, the facilitator distributes the handout **Health Promotion: Promoting Health and Preventing Illness** to the learners. (The facilitator may choose not to distribute the handout if it was recently given to the same learners.)

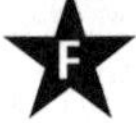 *Today's session is the second of three that comprise the* Pediatrics in Practice *Health Promotion module.*

In today's session, our objectives will be to:

▶ *Discuss a case that will demonstrate how pediatric providers can effectively promote the health of their patients by asking open-ended and follow-up questions*

▶ *Focus on the identification and use of family and community resources*

When we have completed the session, you should be able to answer the following question:

▶ *How can I identify and use family and community resources to promote health and prevent illness?*

The facilitator distributes copies of the case vignette handout **Antoine's 2 Week Visit.**

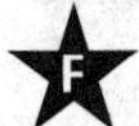 *The child in this case is a 2-week-old breast-feeding baby who is doing well medically. Unless the child health professional looks beyond the initial history and physical exam, the important issues for this family will not be recognized or addressed. Would one of you please read the case aloud for us?*

Discussion and Exercises

The Four-Step Process

1. Identify Relevant Health Promotion Topics

At the display board or flip chart, the facilitator begins the discussion.

 *Can you suggest some examples of open-ended questions you would want to ask Antoine's mother, Celeste?*

After we have created our list, we'll review each question and identify some appropriate follow-up questions.

Examples could include:

▶ Celeste, it's good to see you. Antoine is looking great!

▶ What concerns do you have today?

▶ How do you think breastfeeding is going?

▶ What questions do you have about breastfeeding?

    Follow-up: How often and for how long do you breastfeed?

▶ You seem to be tired, Celeste. Many breastfeeding mothers find that to be the case. Who is able to help you with the baby?

    Follow-up: How often do they help to take care of Antoine?

    Are you able to sleep when he sleeps?

    What do other family members think about your breastfeeding?

▶ How is Antoine's father involved with him?

    Follow-up: What does he like to do with Antoine?

    How does he feel about your breastfeeding?

▶ How do you think that you are holding up?

    Follow-up: Do you find yourself feeling sad?

    Have you been able to get out of the house much?

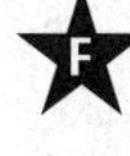 *In cases like this one, you should be very careful and sensitive when asking questions. Some mothers will consider your suggestions to mean that they are not doing well.*

Examples of sensitive questioning include:

▶ What do you plan to do about breastfeeding after you go back to work?

    Follow-up: Are you going to pump your breast milk or supplement with formula?

▶ Many mothers find lactation consultants and mothers from the La Leche League helpful when they are breastfeeding. Would you like to contact someone from either of these groups?

    Follow-up: Are you aware that you can combine breastfeeding and bottle-feeding once breastfeeding is established?

As a refresher, the facilitator might ask learners to compare the characteristics of open-ended interview questions and specific follow-up questions, as in the chart below:

Interview Questions	Directed Follow-up Questions
• Are open ended	• Focus the discussion
• Are nonjudgmental	• Seek specific information
• Allow for follow-up questions	• Can be answered with yes or no

2. Give Personalized Guidance

The facilitator tells the learners that responses to the questions have provided these additional facts:

▶ Celeste is not confident that she is doing a good job with breastfeeding.

▶ Celeste does not feel that she is getting enough support from her husband at home.

▶ Celeste is worried that she won't be able to continue breastfeeding when she goes back to work in a few weeks.

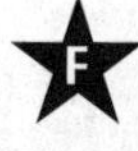 *How would you approach the problems Celeste's responses have revealed (her conflicted feelings about breastfeeding, the involvement of her husband, and her work-related issues)?*

Some possible responses include:

About her feelings concerning breastfeeding:

▶ Reassure her that Antoine's weight gain is excellent and show her the growth chart

▶ Ask her to continue breastfeeding and bring Antoine in for a visit next week

About the father's involvement:

▶ Talk with Celeste about ways to involve the father in Antoine's care

▶ Suggest that the father come in with them at next week's visit

About work-related issues:

▶ Discuss options for finding a time and a place to use a breast pump at work

To enhance the vignette, the facilitator tells the learners that Antoine's father agrees to come to the next visit.

How would you ask Antoine's father about his feelings regarding breastfeeding?

Some possible answers include:

▶ During our prenatal visit, we talked about the changes that a new baby would bring to your lives. Now that Antoine is here, and doing very well, what changes have you noticed most?

▶ How do you think you and Celeste are handling those changes?

▶ Many fathers feel that they are kind of "out of the loop" when a baby is being breastfed. How are you finding life with your new baby?

3. Incorporate Family and Community Resources

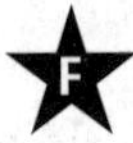

Your questioning has uncovered some concerns about breastfeeding. What community-related resources might you suggest for this family?

Possible answers include:

Workplace:

▶ Recommend that Celeste call her company to ask about breastfeeding arrangements

▶ Encourage her to get the names of other women who have nursed

Community:

▶ Suggest involvement of either a lactation consultant and/or a La Leche instructor

▶ Look for support groups of other mothers who have nursed

If time allows, the facilitator might want to present the following scenario:

You have just moved to a new community. You want to become familiar with the local resources available for the families in your community. What would you do to develop a list of resources?

After some brainstorming, the facilitator should suggest that the learners use their ideas to develop a list for their own clinic, if none exists.

4. Come to Closure with the Family

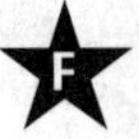

At the end of the health visit, you will want to be sure that the family understands what is being done and what has been decided. What would be a good way to end the health visit?

Some examples might include:

▶ What questions do you have about what we discussed today?

▶ What other concerns do you have about your child's health?

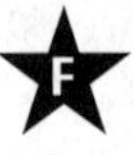

Remember to be alert to any health care barriers that might exist. Barriers such as these can impact the family's ability to follow your guidance.

For example:

▶ Celeste may be unable to use a breast pump at work

▶ Her husband might get angry if he is asked to come to the health visit

Take-Home Message

The facilitator ends the session with the following:

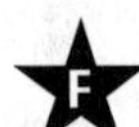

In this session, we have discussed the case of a breastfeeding mother who seemed to be doing well at first glance. Only by asking effective open-ended questions and specific follow-up questions were problems uncovered and resources suggested. Identifying the real needs of each family and using appropriate family and community resources are essential elements in promoting health and preventing illness in your patients. Before we conclude, what questions remain about what we addressed today?

Answers to the Guiding Question

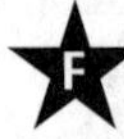

Now that we have completed this session on Health Promotion, you should be able to answer the following question:

▶ How can I identify and use family and community resources to promote health and prevent illness?

  • Become familiar with the child's family and the role of each family member in the care of the child

- Maintain a list of available community resources, including names, phone numbers, and addresses when possible
- Develop working relationships with community professionals and establish lines of referral

Planning for the Next Session (if Session 3 is planned)

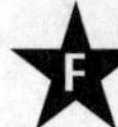 *In our next session, we will perform a reflective exercise based on a health promotion or illness prevention issue that you have encountered. You will have the opportunity to apply the knowledge and skills you have developed in asking interview and follow-up questions, giving personalized guidance, incorporating family and community resources, and coming to closure with the family.*

Evaluation

The facilitator now distributes the **Session Evaluation Form**. The facilitator also completes the **Facilitator Self-Assessment Form.**

Health Promotion: Session 2

HEALTH PROMOTION: PROMOTING HEALTH AND PREVENTING ILLNESS

It is essential that health professionals identify and focus on the individual needs and concerns of the child and family, since families often hesitate to initiate discussion.

1. **Identify relevant health promotion topics.**
   - Ask open-ended, nonjudgmental questions to obtain information and identify appropriate guidance
     Example:
     - *"How is breastfeeding going? What questions/concerns do you have today?"*
   - Ask specific follow-up questions to communicate understanding and focus the discussion
     Example:
     - *"How often and for how long do you breastfeed Manuel? How do you tell when he wants to be fed?"*
   - Listen for verbal and nonverbal cues to discover underlying or unidentified concerns
     Example:
     - *"How do you balance your roles of partner and parent? When do you make time for yourself?"*
     Note:
     - *If parent hesitates with an answer, try to determine the reason.*
     - *If parent brings in child multiple times for minor problems, explore the possibility of another unresolved concern.*

2. **Give personalized guidance.**
   - Introduce new information and reinforce healthy practices
     Examples:
     - *Take time for self, time with partner*
     - *Encourage partner to help care for baby*
     - *Accept support from friends, family*

3. **Incorporate family and community resources.**
   - Approach child within context of family and community
   - Identify each family member's role
     Examples:
     - *"Who helps you with Kim?"*
     - *"How much rest are you getting?"*
   - Identify community resources such as lactation consultant or local La Leche League chapter
   - Develop working relationships with community professionals, and establish lines of referral
   - Create a list of local resources with contact information

4. **Come to closure.**
   - Be sure that the health message is understood
     Examples:
     - *"Have I addressed your concerns?"*
     - *"Do you have any other concerns about Kim's health?"*
   - Identify possible barriers
     Example:
     - *"What problems do you think you might have following through with what we discussed today?"*

Source: Reproduced with permission from Green. M., Palfrey, J.S., Clark, E.M., & Anastasi, J.M. (Eds.) (2002). *Bright futures: Guidelines for health supervision of infants, children, and adolescents* (2nd ed., rev.)—*Pocket guide.* Arlington, VA: National Center for Education in Maternal and Child Health.

Health Promotion: Session 2

CASE VIGNETTE:
ANTOINE'S 2 WEEK VISIT

Antoine is a 2-week-old infant who is brought to your office for a routine health visit. He was born full term, had a normal neonatal course, and had started breastfeeding well prior to discharge on the second day of life. A follow-up phone call to his mother, Celeste, 2 days after discharge indicated that there were no apparent problems. At that time, Antoine seemed to be nursing well. His maternal grandmother was visiting from Chicago and was helping out. Celeste stated that she was getting enough rest.

When you enter the examination room, Celeste is holding Antoine and talking to him. She looks exhausted and seems unhappy. Your examination of Antoine is completely normal. He weighs 10 ounces more than his birth-weight.

Celeste asks about supplementing Antoine's feeding with bottles of formula once or twice a day.

Health Promotion: Session 2

SESSION EVALUATION FORM

Session 2: Asking Questions and Identifying Resources

Date: _______________________________

Facilitator(s): _______________________________

Site: _______________________________

---

1. Overall, I found the "Asking Questions and Identifying Resources" session to be:

Not Useful			Very Useful	
1	2	3	4	5

2. The objectives of the session were:

Not Clear				Clear
1	2	3	4	5

3. The organization of the session was:

Poor				Excellent
1	2	3	4	5

4. The communication skills of the facilitator(s) were:

Poor				Excellent
1	2	3	4	5

5. The facilitator(s) stimulated interest in the subject matter:

Not at All			Very Much	
1	2	3	4	5

6. The facilitator(s) encouraged group participation:

Not at All			Very Much	
1	2	3	4	5

7. Handouts or visual aids (if used) were:

Not Helpful		Very Helpful		
1	2	3	4	5

8. Any additional comments?

____
____
____

9. The most useful features of the session were:

____
____
____

10. Suggestions for improvement

____
____
____

11. Suggestions for topics related to this session

____
____
____

Health Promotion: Session 2

FACILITATOR SELF-ASSESSMENT FORM

Directions: Please rate yourself from 1 to 5 on the following facilitator skills. The closer you are to a 5 within each domain, the more skilled you are at facilitation. We encourage you to complete this form prior to and after each teaching experience (e.g., a single session or an entire module). This will allow you to assess your performance as a facilitator over time.

Facilitator Behavior	1	2	3	4	5
Remains neutral					
Does not judge ideas					
Keeps the group focused on common task					
Asks clarifying questions					
Creates a climate free of criticism					
Encourages participation					
Structures participation					

Source: Adapted with permission from Welch, M. (1999). *Teaching diversity and cultural competence in health care: A trainer's guide.* San Francisco, CA: Perspectives of Differences Diversity Training and Consultation for Health Professionals (PODSDT).

Health Promotion: Session 2

PRECEPTOR STRUCTURED OBSERVATION FORM

Behavior	Observed	Not Observed	Not Applicable
Asked open-ended questions to obtain information			
Followed up with more specific questions			
Communicated understanding to the child and/or family			
Gave personalized guidance and introduced new information			
Identified each family member's role in the care of the child			
Identified community resources if applicable			
Came to closure by making sure that the health message was understood			
Identified and addressed any health care barriers			

Health Promotion: Session 2

LEARNER SELF-ASSESSMENT FORM

During health visits today, I feel that I:	Circle: 1 = disagree to 5 = agree				
Asked open-ended questions to obtain information	1	2	3	4	5
Followed up with more specific questions	1	2	3	4	5
Communicated understanding to the child and/or family	1	2	3	4	5
Gave personalized guidance and introduced new information	1	2	3	4	5
Identified each family member's role in the care of the child	1	2	3	4	5
Identified community resources if applicable	1	2	3	4	5
Came to closure by making sure that the health message was understood	1	2	3	4	5
Identified and addressed any health care barriers	1	2	3	4	5

Health Promotion: Session 2

PATIENT AND FAMILY SURVEY FORM

To our Patients and Families:

The child health professionals in our clinic are very interested in your opinions about the care that we provide for you and your child. As part of our effort to continue to improve the care we offer, we ask that you please complete this survey about today's visit. Your responses will be confidential and will not be shared directly with your child health professional.

Thank you for your time in completing this survey.

The Staff of the Clinic

FAMILY SURVEY Respondent is: ☐ Child ☐ Family					
My Child Health Professional:	Disagree <—> Uncertain <—> Agree				
Addressed the concerns I had about my child	1	2	3	4	5
Listened to me and my child and respected our feelings	1	2	3	4	5
Involved me in decisions	1	2	3	4	5
Talked so that I could understand	1	2	3	4	5
Helped me feel better about my child	1	2	3	4	5
Seemed to care about me and my child	1	2	3	4	5
Gave me adequate time to discuss my concerns	1	2	3	4	5
Provided high-quality care	1	2	3	4	5

Comments

____

____

____

____

____

____

____

____

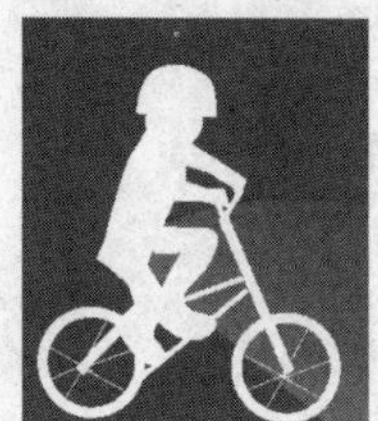

SESSION 3:
A Reflective Exercise

At the beginning of the session, the facilitator and learners should introduce themselves briefly. (If the same group has recently completed Session 2, the facilitator may decide that introductions are not needed.) Ideas for creative introductions can be found in the Facilitator's Guide.

Setting the Context: The Bright Futures Concept

(May be omitted if recently presented or when sessions are combined.)

The facilitator **(F)** introduces the learners to the Bright Futures concept of health by reading or paraphrasing the following:

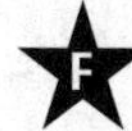 *The World Health Organization has defined health as "a state of complete physical, mental and social well-being and not merely the absence of disease or infirmity." Bright Futures embraces this broad definition of health—one that includes not only prevention of morbidity and mortality, but also the achievement of a child's full potential. In the Bright Futures concept of health, providing the capacity for healthy child development is as important as ameliorating illness or injury. Recognizing and acknowledging the strengths and resources of the child, family, and community are essential to promoting healthy growth and development.*

To build that capacity, the Pediatrics in Practice curriculum focuses on six core concepts: Partnership, Communication, Health Promotion/Illness Prevention, Time Management, Education, and Advocacy. The curriculum also includes a companion module (Health) and videotape that present an overview of Pediatrics in Practice and the Bright Futures approach.

Introducing the Session

Before introducing the session, the facilitator distributes the handout **Health Promotion: Promoting Health and Preventing Illness** to the learners. (The facilitator may choose not to distribute the handout if it was recently given to the same learners.)

 *Today's session is the last of three that comprise the* Pediatrics in Practice *Health Promotion module.*

In today's session, our objectives will be to:

▶ *Reflect on a health promotion or illness prevention issue you have encountered with a child and/or family*

▶ *Apply the knowledge and skills you have developed in asking interview and follow-up questions, giving personalized guidance, incorporating family and community resources, and coming to closure*

▶ *Identify barriers to optimal health care*

Discussion and Exercises

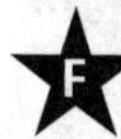 *Today I want you to think about a specific health promotion or illness prevention issue that you have encountered. Topics might include injury prevention, smoking cessation, immunizations, back-to-sleep guidance, or dental referrals. We will discuss one or two of these experiences—keeping in mind effective questioning strategies; personalized guidance; family and community resources; closure and family understanding; and possible solutions to health care barriers.*

Reflective Exercise

The facilitator distributes the **Reflective Exercise** handout and asks learners to:

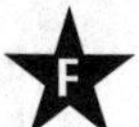 *Take a few minutes to think of the many children and families you have encountered and*

After 2 or 3 minutes, the facilitator should ask the learners to share the topics of their cases. The facilitator should write the topics on a display board or flip chart and ask the learners to choose one or two cases for discussion.

The Four-Step Process

1. Identify Relevant Health Promotion Topics

For each case, the facilitator asks:

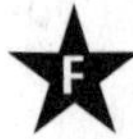 *What are some of the questions you would want to ask in this case?*

Suggestions are recorded on the display board or flip chart.

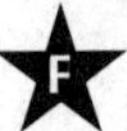 *Let's look at the questions and classify them as either interview or follow-up questions. We also want to discuss why they fit into one category or the other. We will use the chart we have employed in other sessions to compare the questions.*

Interview Questions	Directed Follow-up Questions
• Are open ended	• Focus the discussion
• Are nonjudgmental	• Seek specific information
• Allow for follow-up questions	• Can be answered with yes or no

2. Give Personalized Guidance

For each case, the facilitator asks:

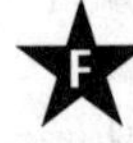 *Can you give some examples of personalized guidance you would provide for the family in this case?*

3. Incorporate Family and Community Resources

The facilitator asks learners to identify family and community resources that could be used in each of the group-selected cases.

 *Can you create a list of specific resources in your community that could be used for the cases we've discussed?*

How would you contact them?

Do you have names of individuals at any of these agencies?

4. Come to Closure with the Family

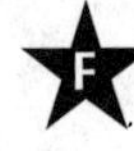 *At the end of the health visit, you will want to be sure that the family has understood the discussions and the recommendations that were made.*

What would be a good way to close the visit?

Examples of questions to ask at the end of the visit are:

▶ Do you have any questions about what we discussed today?

▶ Do you have any other concerns about your child's health?

▶ Do you think you will be able to follow through with what we discussed today?

For each of the cases, the facilitator asks learners to identify and address any barriers that could affect the family's agreement or understanding.

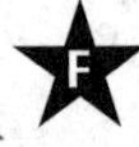 *Can you identify some health care barriers that you've experienced in similar cases? How did you overcome them or try to overcome them?*

If the learners do not readily come up with barriers, some examples and solutions are listed on the table on the next page to initiate the discussion:

Alternative to Reflective Exercise

Two prepared case vignettes may be used if the reflective exercise (which is preferred) is not chosen. The facilitator can use the same steps as those in the activities for cases emerging from the reflective exercise.

Take-Home Message

The facilitator ends the session with the following:

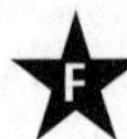 *During this session, we have discussed the skills you will need in promoting health and preventing illness with the children and families you encounter each day. We have practiced formulating effective open-ended and specific follow-up questions and providing personalized guidance. We have also*

explored ways to include family and community resources in comprehensive care.

As child health professionals, we recognize that we must ensure that families understand our discussions and recommendations. By identifying and overcoming potential health care barriers, we can fulfill our unique capacity to promote health and prevent illness.

Before we conclude, what questions remain about what we addressed today?

Evaluation

The facilitator now distributes the **Session Evaluation Form**. The facilitator also completes the **Facilitator Self-Assessment Form**.

Barrier	Possible Solution
Health Professional Related	
Lack of family trust	Ask parents to return more often for routine follow-up visits
	Use good interview techniques, and ask parent to share his/her concerns
Lack of confidence in the role of child health professional	Observe behavior of senior health professionals
	Observe more experienced learners and ask them for suggestions
Lack of staff development (receptionist, etc.)	Have regular staff meetings
	Ask for staff suggestions for change and follow through with suggestions
Limited time spent with patient	Organize schedule to allow for sufficient time with each patient
	Never appear to be hurried, and ask open-ended questions even when rushed
Family Related	
Fear, anxiety, denial, lack of information	Use open-ended questions to identify needs and address them
Lack of resources	Involve social and community services
Parent and/or grandparent discord	Suggest family conferences Invite grandparents to next visit
Community Related	
Hospital policy not "baby-friendly" (e.g., doesn't promote breastfeeding)	Become involved in hospital administration
	Encourage families to participate on hospital's-community board
Difficulty in contacting the appropriate personnel in social service agencies	Help families and agencies connect

Health Promotion: Session 3

HEALTH PROMOTION: PROMOTING HEALTH AND PREVENTING ILLNESS

It is essential that health professionals identify and focus on the individual needs and concerns of the child and family, since families often hesitate to initiate discussion.

1. Identify relevant health promotion topics.

- Ask open-ended, nonjudgmental questions to obtain information and identify appropriate guidance
  Example:
  - *"How is breastfeeding going? What questions/concerns do you have today?"*
- Ask specific follow-up questions to communicate understanding and focus the discussion
  Example:
  - *"How often and for how long do you breastfeed Manuel? How do you tell when he wants to be fed?"*
- Listen for verbal and nonverbal cues to discover underlying or unidentified concerns
  Example:
  - *"How do you balance your roles of partner and parent? When do you make time for yourself?"*
  Note:
  - *If parent hesitates with an answer, try to determine the reason.*
  - *If parent brings in child multiple times for minor problems, explore the possibility of another unresolved concern.*

2. Give personalized guidance.

- Introduce new information and reinforce healthy practices
  Examples:
  - *Take time for self, time with partner*
  - *Encourage partner to help care for baby*
  - *Accept support from friends, family*

3. Incorporate family and community resources.

- Approach child within context of family and community
- Identify each family member's role
  Examples:
  - *"Who helps you with Kim?"*
  - *"How much rest are you getting?"*
- Identify community resources such as lactation consultant or local La Leche League chapter
- Develop working relationships with community professionals, and establish lines of referral
- Create a list of local resources with contact information

4. Come to closure.

- Be sure that the health message is understood
  Examples:
  - *"Have I addressed your concerns?"*
  - *"Do you have any other concerns about Kim's health?"*
- Identify possible barriers
  Example:
  - *"What problems do you think you might have following through with what we discussed today?"*

Source: Reproduced with permission from Green. M., Palfrey, J.S., Clark, E.M., & Anastasi, J.M. (Eds.) (2002). *Bright futures: Guidelines for health supervision of infants, children, and adolescents* (2nd ed., rev.)—*Pocket guide.* Arlington, VA: National Center for Education in Maternal and Child Health.

Health Promotion: Session 3

REFLECTIVE EXERCISE

Take a few minutes to think of the many patients you have encountered and the various health promotion and illness prevention issues they have revealed to you. Narrow your focus to one or two cases that you remember as being particularly outstanding. Try to summarize the case in three sentences or so. If you wish, you can discuss your case with the person sitting next to you.

Health Promotion: Session 3

ALTERNATE CASE VIGNETTES

Alternate Case 1

An 8-year-old girl comes in for a routine health assessment. She states that she is doing well, and she has no physical complaints.

Alternate Case 2

A 15-year-old male comes in for a routine health assessment. He looks upset, does not smile, and tells you that he doesn't want to be there.

Health Promotion: Session 3

SESSION EVALUATION FORM

Session 3: A Reflective Exercise

Date: _______________________________

Facilitator(s): _______________________________

Site: _______________________________

---

1. Overall, I found the "Reflective Exercise" session to be:

Not Useful				Very Useful
1	2	3	4	5

2. The objectives of the session were:

Not Clear				Clear
1	2	3	4	5

3. The organization of the session was:

Poor				Excellent
1	2	3	4	5

4. The communication skills of the facilitator(s) were:

Poor				Excellent
1	2	3	4	5

5. The facilitator(s) stimulated interest in the subject matter:

Not at All				Very Much
1	2	3	4	5

6. The facilitator(s) encouraged group participation:

Not at All				Very Much
1	2	3	4	5

7. Handouts or visual aids (if used) were:

Not Helpful				Very Helpful
1	2	3	4	5

8. Any additional comments?

____

____

____

9. The most useful features of the session were:

____

____

____

10. Suggestions for improvement

____

____

____

11. Suggestions for topics related to this session

____

____

Health Promotion: Session 3

FACILITATOR SELF-ASSESSMENT FORM

Directions: Please rate yourself from 1 to 5 on the following facilitator skills. The closer you are to a 5 within each domain, the more skilled you are at facilitation. We encourage you to complete this form prior to and after each teaching experience (e.g., a single session or an entire module). This will allow you to assess your performance as a facilitator over time.

Facilitator Behavior	1	2	3	4	5
Remains neutral					
Does not judge ideas					
Keeps the group focused on common task					
Asks clarifying questions					
Creates a climate free of criticism					
Encourages participation					
Structures participation					

Source: Adapted with permission from Welch, M. (1999). *Teaching diversity and cultural competence in health care: A trainer's guide.* San Francisco, CA: Perspectives of Differences Diversity Training and Consultation for Health Professionals (PODSDT).

Health Promotion: Session 3

PRECEPTOR STRUCTURED OBSERVATION FORM

Behavior	Observed	Not Observed	Not Applicable
Asked open-ended questions to obtain information			
Followed up with more specific questions			
Communicated understanding to the child and/or family			
Gave personalized guidance and introduced new information			
Identified each family member's role in the care of the child			
Identified community resources if applicable			
Came to closure by making sure that the health message was understood			
Identified and addressed any health care barriers			

Health Promotion: Session 3

LEARNER SELF-ASSESSMENT FORM

During health visits today, I feel that I:	Circle: 1=disagree to 5=agree				
Asked open-ended questions to obtain information	1	2	3	4	5
Followed up with more specific questions	1	2	3	4	5
Communicated understanding to the child and/or family	1	2	3	4	5
Gave personalized guidance and introduced new information	1	2	3	4	5
Identified each family member's role in the care of the child	1	2	3	4	5
Identified community resources if applicable	1	2	3	4	5
Came to closure by making sure that the health message was understood	1	2	3	4	5
Identified and addressed any health care barriers	1	2	3	4	5

Health Promotion: Session 3

PATIENT AND FAMILY SURVEY FORM

To our Patients and Families:

The child health professionals in our clinic are very interested in your opinions about the care that we provide for you and your child. As part of our effort to continue to improve the care we offer, we ask that you please complete this survey about today's visit. Your responses will be confidential and will not be shared directly with your child health professional.

Thank you for your time in completing this survey.

The Staff of the Clinic

FAMILY SURVEY	Respondent is: ☐ Child ☐ Family				
My Child Health Professional:	Disagree <—> Uncertain <—> Agree				
Addressed the concerns I had about my child	1	2	3	4	5
Listened to me and my child and respected our feelings	1	2	3	4	5
Involved me in decisions	1	2	3	4	5
Talked so that I could understand	1	2	3	4	5
Helped me feel better about my child	1	2	3	4	5
Seemed to care about me and my child	1	2	3	4	5
Gave me adequate time to discuss my concerns	1	2	3	4	5
Provided high-quality care	1	2	3	4	5

Comments

____

____

____

____

____

____

____

References

Benjamin, J.T., Cimino, S.A., & Hafler, J.P., Bright Futures Health Promotion Work Group, & Bernstein, H.H. (2002). The office visit: A time to promote health—but how? *Contemporary Pediatrics, 19*(2), 90–107.

Breslow, L. (1999). From disease prevention to health promotion. *JAMA, 281*(11), 1030–1033.

Cheng, T.L., Greenberg, L., Loeser, H., & Keller, D. (2000). Teaching prevention in pediatrics. *Academic Medicine, 75,* 866–871.

Cordes, D.H., Rea, D.F., Kligman, E., & Eichling, P. (1995). Meanwhile back at the ranch: Training residents in clinical preventive medicine. *American Journal of Preventive Medicine, 11*(3), 145–148.

Green, M. (1995). No child is an island: Contextual pediatrics and the "new" health supervision. *Pediatric Clinics of North America, 42*(1), 79–87.

Green, M., & Palfrey, J.S. (Eds.) (2002). *Bright futures: Guidelines for health supervision of infants, children, and adolescents* (2nd ed., rev.). Arlington, VA: National Center for Education in Maternal and Child Health.

Green, M., Palfrey, J.S., Clark, E.M., & Anastasi, J.M. (Eds.) (2002). *Bright futures: Guidelines for health supervision of infants, children, and adolescents* (2nd ed., rev.)—*Pocket guide.* Arlington, VA: National Center for Education in Maternal and Child Health.

Hwang, M.Y. (1999). How to talk with your doctor. *JAMA, 282*(24), 2422.

Keim, D.B., Gomez, C.F., & Wolf, A.M.D. (1998). The level of preventive health care in an internal medicine residency clinic: Still only an ounce of prevention? *Southern Medical Journal, 91*(6), 550–554.

Lane, D.S. (1992). Developing primary care curricula in preventive medicine: Some practical considerations. *American Journal of Preventive Medicine, 8*(6), 389–394.

Nutting, P.A. (1986). Health promotion in primary medical care: Problems and potential. *Preventive Medicine, 15,* 537–548.

Palfrey, J.S. (1997). Keeping children and families in the center of our concern. *Archives of Pediatrics and Adolescent Medicine, 151,* 337–340.

Palfrey, J.S. (1998). Comprehensive child health: Is it in the picture? *Archives of Pediatrics and Adolescent Medicine, 152,* 222–223.

Resources

Adult Learning Principles and Clinical Teaching

Roberts, K.B. (1996). Educational principles of community-based education. *Pediatrics* (Suppl., Dec. 1996)98:1259–1263.

Spencer, P.E., & Alden, E. (1996). Educational foundations for community-based programs. In DeWitt, T., & Roberts, K. (Eds.), *Pediatric education in community settings: A manual* (p. 14). Arlington, VA: National Center for Education in Maternal and Child Health.

Whitman, N., & Schwenk, T. (1997). *The physician as teacher* (2nd ed., pp. 33–37). Salt Lake City, UT: Whitman Associates.

Other Clinical Teaching Models (similar to the "Teachable Moments" model)

McGee, S.R., & Irby, D.M. (1997). Teaching in the outpatient clinic: Practical tips. *Journal of general Internal Medicine, 12,* S34–S40.

Neher, G., & Meyer, S. (1992). A five-step microskills model of clinical teaching. *Journal of the American Board of Family Practice, 5,* 419–424.

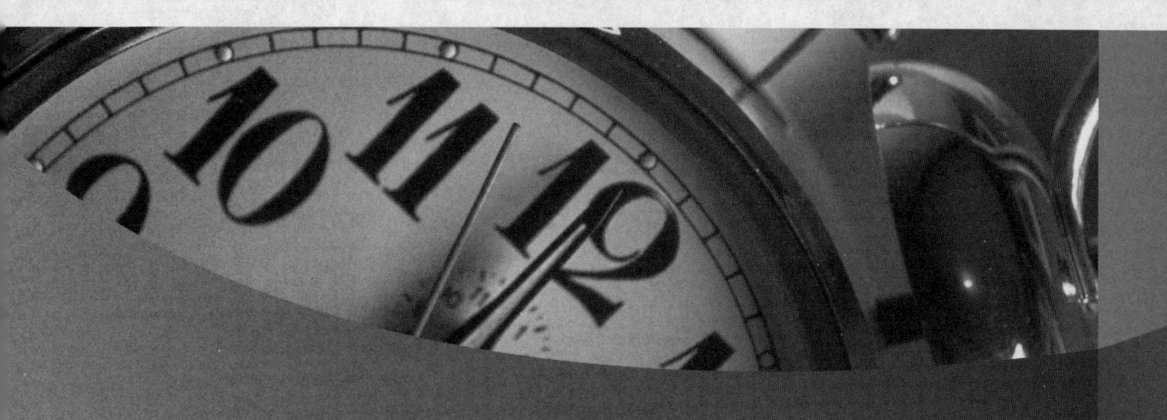

Chapter 6

Time Management

Managing Time for Health Promotion

Franklin Trimm

Joe Lopreiato

CONTENTS

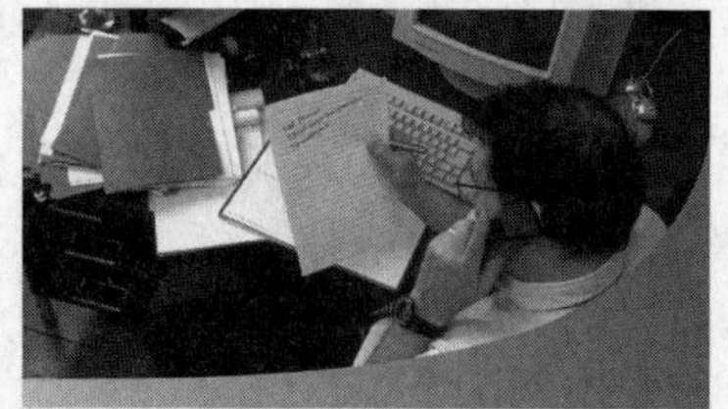

TIME MANAGEMENT
Managing Time for Health Promotion

OVERVIEW

Background

Today's health professionals face intense pressures to provide health care for increasing numbers of children and their families, including many with complex medical and behavioral problems. The American Academy of Pediatrics, the Centers for Disease Control and Prevention, the U.S. Preventive Services Task Force, Bright Futures, and others have recommended providing expanded health promotion and preventive services to meet these challenges. Yet, the average time for a pediatric health visit remains approximately 15 minutes. In today's health care environment, time management skills are essential tools for providing effective health supervision.

Goals

The goal of this module is to enhance health promotion through teaching a five-step model for integrating effective time management techniques into health supervision.

This module will enable learners to:

▶ Apply the five-step Time Management Model to manage the health visit more efficiently

▶ Acquire the knowledge and skills to prioritize goals for the health visit

▶ Understand the role of collaboration and partnership when setting priorities for the health visit

▶ Use the *Bright Futures Encounter Forms for Families* as a time management tool to identify family needs and concerns, help the family prepare for the health visit, and provide guidance on important health topics

▶ Become familiar with the American Academy of Pediatrics' *Well Child Visit Documentation Forms* as an effective time management tool

▶ Explore the use of health promotion packets in enhancing the health visit

Instructional Design

This module consists of two 30-minute sessions:

▶ Session 1 presents the five-step Time Management Model and provides opportunities to apply these steps, based on a case vignette.

▶ Session 2 examines the use of family encounter forms and pediatric visit documentation forms as effective time management tools for the health visit.

▶ Each of the two sessions can be used as a separate, stand-alone offering, or the sessions can be combined. See the Facilitator's Guide for information on combining sessions.

Teaching Strategies

The teaching strategies used in this module include case discussion and brainstorming. These strategies have been selected to help learners understand and apply the five-step Time Management Model in their health encounters with children and families. Please refer to the Facilitator's Guide for more information related to each strategy.

Evaluation

Learners will complete a **Session Evaluation Form** following each session. Facilitators are encouraged to complete a **Facilitator Self-**

Assessment Form prior to and following each teaching experience (e.g., a single session or an entire module) in order to assess their performance over time.

Guiding Questions

Learners who have completed the entire Time Management module should be able to answer the following questions:

▶ How can I deliver enhanced health promotion services in a timely manner consistent with the real-world demands of pediatric health care, including care for children with medically and socially complex needs?

▶ How do core concepts and skills such as building a partnership with the family improve the efficiency of providing health promotion services? Improve time management?

▶ How do interview questions improve the efficiency of the health visit?

▶ How can Bright Futures and other health promotion materials help make health visits more efficient?

▶ What strategies can minimize the time spent filling out forms to document the visit?

INTRODUCTION TO TEACHING SESSIONS

Session 1: Applying the Five-Step Time Management Model

Objectives

The objectives for this session are for the facilitator to:

▶ Present the five-step Time Management Model for managing the health visit more efficiently

▶ Help learners acquire the knowledge and skills to prioritize goals for the health visit

▶ Help learners understand the role of collaboration and partnership when setting priorities for the health visit

Materials

The materials and teaching aids needed for this session are:

Handouts

▶ Time Management: Managing Time for Health Promotion

▶ Initial Self-Assessment of Time Management

▶ Case Vignette: Jacob's 4 Month Visit, Part 1

▶ Case Vignette: Jacob's 4 Month Visit, Part 2

▶ Bright Futures 4 Month Visit, Questions for the Parent(s)

▶ Follow-Up Self-Assessment of Time Management

▶ Session Evaluation Form

Facilitator Form

▶ Facilitator Self-Assessment Form

Teaching Aids

▶ Display board, flip chart, or chalkboard

▶ Markers or chalk

Time

The time allocated for this session is 30 minutes.

Session 2: Using Encounter and Documentation Forms As Time Management Tools

Objectives

The objectives for this session are for the facilitator to:

▶ Demonstrate how *Bright Futures Encounter Forms for Families* serve as a time management tool to identify family needs and concerns, help the family prepare for the health visit, and provide guidance on important health topics

▶ Introduce the American Academy of Pediatrics' *Well Child Visit Documentation Forms* as an effective time management tool

▶ Emphasize the use of health promotion packets in enhancing the health visit

Materials

The materials and teaching aids needed for this session are:

Handouts

▶ Time Management: Managing Time for Health Promotion

▶ Bright Futures Encounter Forms for Families: 4 Month Visit

▶ American Academy of Pediatrics Well Child/4 Months Visit Documentation Form

▶ Session Evaluation Form

Facilitator Form

▶ Facilitator Self-Assessment Form

Teaching Aids

▶ Display board, flip chart, or chalkboard

▶ Markers or chalk

Time

The time allocated for this session is 30 minutes.

SESSION 1:
Applying the Five-Step Time Management Model

At the beginning of the session, the facilitator and learners should introduce themselves briefly. Ideas for creative introductions can be found in the Facilitator's Guide.

Setting the Context: The Bright Futures Concept

The facilitator (**F**) introduces the learners to the Bright Futures concept of health by reading or paraphrasing the following:

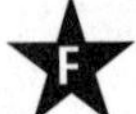

The World Health Organization has defined health as "a state of complete physical, mental and social well-being and not merely the absence of disease or infirmity." Bright Futures embraces this broad definition of health—one that includes not only prevention of morbidity and mortality, but also the achievement of a child's full potential. In the Bright Futures concept of health, providing the capacity for healthy child development is as important as ameliorating illness or injury. Recognizing and acknowledging the strengths and resources of the child, family, and community are essential to promoting healthy growth and development.

To build that capacity, the Pediatrics in Practice curriculum focuses on six core concepts: Partnership, Communication, Health Promotion/Illness Prevention, Time Management, Education, and Advocacy. The curriculum also includes a companion module (Health) and videotape that present an overview of Pediatrics in Practice and the Bright Futures approach.

Introducing the Session

Before introducing the session, the facilitator distributes the handout **Time Management: Managing Time for Health Promotion.**

This session is the first of two that comprise the Pediatrics in Practice *Time Management*

module. In today's complex health care environment, time management skills have become indispensable tools for health promotion.

Today's health professionals face intense pressures to provide health care for increasing numbers of children and their families, including many with complex medical and behavioral problems. The American Academy of Pediatrics, the Centers for Disease Control and Prevention, the U.S. Preventive Services Task Force, Bright Futures, and others recommend expanded health promotion and preventive services to meet these challenges. Yet, the average time for a pediatric health visit is only 14.2 minutes.

In this session, we will discuss an approach or model for managing the limited time available, in order to accomplish as many goals as possible during the health visit.

In today's session, our objectives will be to:

▶ *Learn the five-step Time Management Model to manage the health visit more efficiently*

▶ *Acquire the knowledge and skills to prioritize goals for the health visit*

▶ *Understand the role of collaboration and partnership when setting priorities for the health visit*

When we have completed the session, you should be able to answer the following questions:

▶ *How can I deliver enhanced health promotion services in a timely manner consistent with the real-world demands of pediatric health care, including care for children with medically and socially complex needs?*

▶ *How do core concepts and skills such as building a partnership with the family improve the efficiency of providing health promotion services? Improve time management?*

► *How do interview questions improve the efficiency of the health visit?*

Discussion and Exercises

Initial Self-Assessment Exercise

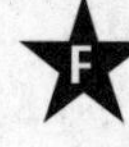 *Before we begin, I am going to distribute copies of the handout **Initial Self-Assessment of Time Management**. Take 2 or 3 minutes to think about how frequently you use some of these time management tools. (This exercise is for your own personal use; it will not be collected.)*

The facilitator initiates a brief discussion on the self-assessment exercise, using one of the following questions:

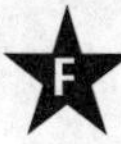 *Looking at your self-assessment, let's talk about areas where we could become more time-efficient.*

or:

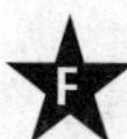 *Looking at your self-assessment, what areas seem to be most challenging for you? Why?*

Applying the Five-Step Time Management Model

The facilitator then reads or paraphrases the following:

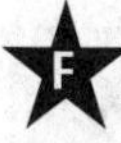 *Time management helps us to use time in the most effective and productive way possible. The Time Management Model consists of five essential steps:*

1. Maximize time for health promotion (by minimizing documentation time)

2. Clarify the health professional's goals for the visit

3. Identify the family's needs and concerns for the visit

4. Work with the family to prioritize goals for the visit

5. Suggest other options for addressing unmet goals

We are now going to apply this model step by step, based on the case of Jacob Downing and his mother, who have come to the clinic for Jacob's 4 month visit.

The facilitator distributes the handout **Case Vignette: Jacob's 4 Month Visit, Part 1** and asks one of the learners to read it aloud.

Maximizing Time for Health Promotion

After a learner reads the handout aloud, the facilitator reads or paraphrases:

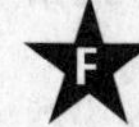 *The focus of this discussion is the implementation of each step of the model. Step 1 of the Time Management Model is to maximize time for health promotion. This can be accomplished through a range of techniques, such as using checklists and standardized documentation forms. What strategies would you, as a pediatric provider, use to minimize the time spent documenting Jacob's health visit in order to have more time to discuss the family's health concerns?*

Learners' responses might include the following:

► Use accurate screening and record-keeping forms to reduce documentation time.

► Ask Jacob's mother to complete standard screening forms while in the waiting room. (Bright Futures Encounter Forms for Families—described in the next session—not only help explain what happens during the visit but also help identify some of the family's health concerns.)

► Organize charts consistently for all of Jacob's health visits, to track and retrieve information easily.

► Scan or review Jacob's chart before meeting with the family.

► Train office staff to document basic information (e.g., Jacob's feeding and sleeping habits, immunization status) and to provide follow-up with the family.

► Combine tasks (e.g., provide some anticipatory guidance while doing the physical exam).

Clarifying the Health Professional's Goals for the Visit

The facilitator moves to the display board, draws a line down the middle to create two columns, labels the first column "Health Professional's Goals," then opens the discussion.

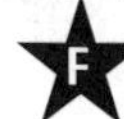 *Step 2 of the Time Management Model is to clarify the health professional's goals for the visit. As professionals, we enter into each health visit with an agenda. We must become fully aware of our own goals as well as the family's goals for a health encounter*

before attempting to set priorities for the health visit. Being fully aware of this agenda is a vital step in managing health visits efficiently. In addition to completing the physical exam and necessary screening and immunizations, what goals do you, as Jacob's pediatric provider, have for this 4 month health visit?

The facilitator writes down the goals offered by the learners. The list might include:

▶ Promoting specific Bright Futures guidance for the 4 month visit

- *Healthy and safe habits:* Use car seat, put baby to sleep on back, childproof home, keep one hand on baby in high places, introduce solid foods, other topics (additional Bright Futures guidance)

- *Parent-infant interaction:* Hold, cuddle, rock baby; talk, sing, read, play music, use games and toys; keep bedtime routine, use comfort objects

- *Family relationships:* Take time for self and with partner, involve family in baby's care, maintain contact with friends and family (see also maternal needs/coping)

- *Community interaction:* Provide referrals; recommend play and parent support groups, community involvement

▶ Maternal needs and coping skills

▶ How to avoid getting farther behind in seeing patients

[Note to facilitator: Try to elicit a substantive list of goals to emphasize how much could be accomplished during the visit and to identify which items are reasonable to address (by setting priorities). Later in the exercise, this list forms the basis for comparing common concerns and differences between the health professional's and the family's goals, and for discussing how best to collaborate with the family to develop a realistic agenda.]

If necessary, the facilitator prompts discussion by asking additional questions:

What healthy and safe habits do you think should be addressed at a 4 month health visit?

What parent/infant interaction behaviors would you want this mother to know?

What aspects of the family relationships would be important to address?

After the initial list of health professional's goals has been completed, the facilitator reads or paraphrases:

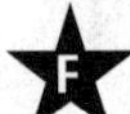

This list appears to have a lot in common with a menu in a restaurant. There are many good things to choose from, but no way to have them all. Bright Futures questions for parents also offer a "menu" from which the health professional can select the questions most appropriate for an individual child and family. Skillful use of these interview questions can help identify both the professional's and the family's goals for the health visit.

The facilitator distributes the handout **Bright Futures 4 Month Visit: Questions for the Parent(s)** and focuses on the role of interview questions in establishing or clarifying goals and concerns for the health visit.

Identifying the Family's Needs and Concerns for the Visit

The facilitator reads or paraphrases:

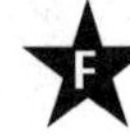

Step 3 of the model is to identify the family's needs or concerns for the visit. Too often, pediatric providers hesitate to identify all of the family's health concerns for fear of getting farther behind in their schedule (like Jacob's provider in the case we just read). Identifying the family's goals and concerns for the health visit is a vital step in managing health promotion efficiently. How can you, as a pediatric provider, identify what the mother's goals might be for this visit?

Learners' responses might include the following:

▶ Begin by asking family-friendly, open-ended, general questions, such as:

- "How are you today? How are things going in your family?"

- "What is your day with Jacob like?"

- "What do you enjoy most about Jacob?"

- "What new things are you seeing Jacob do?"

▶ Follow up with specific Bright Futures interview questions for the 4 month visit, such as:

- "How is feeding going? What do you feed Jacob?"

- "Tell me about Jacob's sleeping habits. Do you put him to sleep on his back?"

- "What questions or concerns do you have about Jacob?"
- "How do you know what Jacob needs or wants. Is it easy or difficult to tell?"
- "What have you found to be the best way to comfort him?"

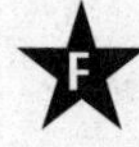 *Bright Futures materials offer a variety of open-ended and focused interview questions that are appropriate for each recommended health visit. These questions are designed to help elicit concerns and engage the family as active partners in the visit.*

The facilitator distributes the handout **Case Vignette: Jacob's 4 Month Visit, Part 2**, asks one of the learners to read it aloud, then opens the discussion.

 *Now that we have identified some of the interview questions that might be particularly relevant for the Downing family, let's continue with the case. In Part 2, the health professional learns more about the family through skillful use of interview questions.*

Based on what you have learned from the interview questions, what needs or concerns do you think Jacob's mother has?

The facilitator labels the second column "Family's Goals or Concerns" and lists the learners' responses, which might include:

▶ Adequacy and confidence in parenting

▶ Colic/irritability

▶ Sleep problems

▶ Relationship between mother and grand-mother

▶ Concerns about whether Jacob's development seems "normal"

▶ Concerns about whether Jacob may be ill

If necessary, the facilitator prompts discussion by asking the following question:

Do you think that Eileen has any concerns about ______________? [*Note to facilitator:* Use any items on the list above.]

Reaching a Common Agenda— Working with the Family to Prioritize Goals for the Visit

After the learners have identified a list of family goals and concerns, the facilitator continues:

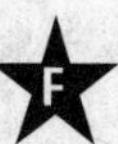 *Now we have two menus—one for the health professional and one for the family. Step 4 of our model is to work with the family to prioritize goals for the visit. Differences in priorities between the health professional's and family's menus can create interactions that are ineffective, inefficient, and frustrating for both the health professional and the family. Collaborating with the family in choosing and prioritizing which items get addressed can make the visit more effective*

The facilitator poses the following question and invites discussion to clarify how to prioritize items on the agenda:

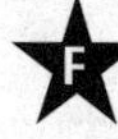 *How would you go about developing a realistic agenda that meets Eileen's and Jacob's needs as well as your own priorities?*

The facilitator writes down the learners' responses, which might include the following:

▶ Explain that the purpose of the health visit is to identify and address the family's specific concerns, and to promote Jacob's healthy growth and development.

▶ Identify the agenda items shared by both the family and the health professional.

▶ Prioritize identified concerns through family-friendly negotiation.

Example: "There are several things about Jacob we could discuss today. What would be most helpful for us to talk about?"

Example: "I appreciate your concerns about ________. While you are here, can we also talk about ________?"

▶ Prioritize the specific medical and health promotion concepts for the 4 month visit that are most relevant to Jacob and his mother (e.g., addressing Jacob's feeding and sleeping habits, helping Eileen gain confidence in her parenting skills). Some health promotion concepts may need to be addressed in a separate visit or follow-up phone call if the family's needs warrant.

[*Note to facilitator:* If learners need prompting in generating responses similar to those above, offer one or two sample responses to elicit suggestions. Validate any suggestions offered, because there are many ways to build consensus between the family and the health professional.]

Health Professional's Goals	Family's Goals or Concerns
Promoting specific guidance for the 4 month visit	Adequacy and confidence in parenting
• Healthy and safe habits: car seat, sleep on back, childproof home, infant safety, solid foods, other Bright Futures topics	• Colic/irritability • Sleep problems • Is Jacob ill? • Is Jacob's development "normal"?
• Parent/infant interaction: hold, cuddle, rock, talk, sing, read, play; bedtime routine, comfort objects	Ways to soothe Jacob when he is fussy or colicky
• Family relationships: time for self and partner, involvement of family in baby's care, contact with friends and family	Relationship between mother and grandmother
• Community interaction: referrals, play and parent support groups, community involvement	Additional help or support with maternal coping skills
How to avoid getting farther behind in seeing patients	

Suggesting Other Options for Addressing Unmet Goals

The facilitator introduces the fifth step in the Time Management Model and asks learners to suggest ways to address goals that could not be met during the visit.

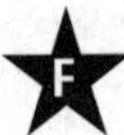 *Identifying and prioritizing goals and reaching a common agenda are important steps. The fifth and final step in our Time Management Model is to suggest other options for addressing unmet goals. Be sure to validate all of the family's goals, even those that could not be addressed during the health visit. What are some resources the health professional might use to deal with these unmet needs or concerns?*

Learners' responses might include:

▶ Educational materials (print, audio, video, Internet)

▶ Follow-up visits or phone calls

▶ Referrals to other professional or community resources

Take-Home Message

The facilitator reads or paraphrases:

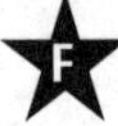 *This teaching session was based on a five-step model for managing time more efficiently during the health visit.*

In summary, these are the five steps:

▶ *Maximize time for health promotion*

▶ *Clarify the health professional's goals for the visit*

▶ *Identify the family's needs and concerns for the visit*

▶ *Work with the family to prioritize goals for the visit*

▶ *Suggest other options for addressing unmet goals*

In today's session we've applied these steps to

a case vignette as a practical way to build time management skills in the context of health encounters. Before we conclude, what questions remain about what we addressed today?

In concluding the session, the facilitator distributes the handout **Follow-Up Self-Assessment of Time Management** and states:

In clinical practice, this self-assessment can help you gauge your use of the time management techniques we've been discussing. This process of self-evaluation will help you remember to incorporate and actively practice these steps in health encounters with families. You might also find it helpful to list any barriers on the back of the self-assessment form.

Optional Discussion

If time permits and discussion is of interest to the group, the facilitator asks:

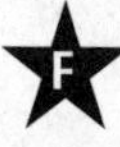

What would you do differently if the mother's anger over being kept waiting so long presented a barrier to an effective visit?

Sample responses might include:

▶ Apologize for keeping Jacob's mother waiting (e.g., "I'm so sorry that I'm late and have kept you waiting—there was an emergency in the neonatal ICU").

▶ Recognize the importance of her time (e.g., consider discounting the cost of the visit if there are out-of-pocket expenses for the mother).

▶ Reassure her that you are going to spend time with her and address her concerns now that you are there (e.g., sit down, assume relaxed posture, don't forego common courtesies).

▶ Move into collaboration as early as possible to demonstrate that the mother's concerns will be addressed.

Answers to the Guiding Questions

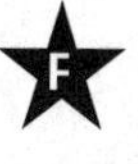

Now that we have completed this session on Time Management, you should be able to answer the following questions:

▶ How can I deliver enhanced health promotion services in a timely manner consistent with the real-world demands of pediatric health care, including care for children with medically and socially complex needs?

• Enhanced health promotion services can be delivered by incorporating the five steps of the Time Management Model:

1. Maximize time for health promotion

2. Clarify the health professional's goals for the visit

3. Identify the family's needs and concerns for the visit

4. Work with the family to prioritize goals for the visit

5. Suggest other options for addressing unmet goals

▶ How do core concepts and skills such as building a partnership with the family improve the efficiency of providing health promotion services? Improve time management?

• Partnership ensures that the highest-priority concerns for the child's health are addressed in the time available, while lower-priority concerns are met through other methods (handouts, Internet resources, follow-up phone calls, referrals).

• When families and pediatric providers work together toward the same goals, mutual trust will develop and any differences of opinion can be resolved more quickly.

• An effective health partnership helps the family better prepare for the health visit by anticipating and providing the information needed (interval history, health habits, special concerns), thus minimizing the time required for the provider to gather this information.

▶ How do interview questions improve the efficiency of the health visit?

• Interview questions help make the health visit more efficient by:

Guiding the family into a discussion about their child's health and their health promotion needs.

Facilitating the family's meaningful participation in the health visit.

Guiding the pediatric provider in addressing age-specific pertinent health topics for the visit.

Planning for the Next Session
(if Session 2 is planned)

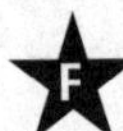

In the next session, we will use encounter forms and documentation forms to illustrate how such tools can enhance health promotion by minimizing the time needed to document the health visit.

To prepare for the next session, the facilitator asks the learners to consider the following questions:

▶ What Bright Futures or other health promotion materials might be useful in making health visits more efficient?

▶ What strategies or techniques have you used to minimize the amount of time spent filling out forms to document the visit?

Evaluation

The facilitator now distributes the **Session Evaluation Form**. The facilitator also completes the **Facilitator Self-Assessment Form**.

Time Management: Session 1

TIME MANAGEMENT: MANAGING TIME FOR HEALTH PROMOTION

1. Maximize time for health promotion.
- Use accurate methods that minimize documentation time
- Ask family to complete forms in waiting area
- Organize chart in consistent manner
- Scan chart before meeting with the child and family
- Train staff to elicit information and to provide follow-up with family

2. Clarify health professional's goals for visit.
- Review screening forms and other basic health data
- Observe parent-infant interaction
- Clarify key issues for visit
  Example: Review age-appropriate anticipatory guidance.
- Identify needs, then rank them in order of importance

3. Identify family's needs and concerns for visit.
- Selectively use Bright Futures general and age-appropriate interview questions
- Include open-ended questions to draw family into visit
  Example: "Tell me about Sabrina's sleeping habits. What position does she sleep in?" (Elicits more than yes/no answer, and presents "teachable moment" on "Back to Sleep" and SIDS.)

4. Work with the family to prioritize goals for visit.
- Explain purpose of visit (identify, address specific concerns and overall health and development)
- Identify family's and health professional's shared goals
- Prioritize needs through family-friendly negotiation
  Example: "I appreciate your concerns about _______. While you are here, I would also like to talk about _______."

5. Suggest other options for addressing unmet goals.
- Acknowledge importance of issues that could not be fully addressed during the visit
- Offer additional resources (handouts, audiotapes, videotapes, Web-based materials)
- Suggest a follow-up visit or phone call
  Example: "I'm sorry we weren't able to talk about _______ during today's visit. Could I call you one afternoon next week to follow up on that?"
  Or: "Would you be able to come back next week so we could talk more about that?"
- Provide referral to professional or community resource
  Example: "I know we haven't had a chance to cover your concern about _______ today. Would you like to pursue it with a specialist in that area?"

Source: Reproduced with permission from Green. M., Palfrey, J.S., Clark, E.M., & Anastasi, J.M. (Eds.) (2002). *Bright futures: Guidelines for health supervision of infants, children, and adolescents* (2nd ed., rev.)—*Pocket guide.* Arlington, VA: National Center for Education in Maternal and Child Health.

Time Management: Session 1

INITIAL SELF-ASSESSMENT OF TIME MANAGEMENT

Question: How often do you use the following time management techniques in your clinical practice?

Time Management Techniques	Frequency of Use			
	Almost Never	**Sometimes**	**Frequently**	**Always**
Use record-keeping methods that keep accurate documentation time to a minimum				
Clarify health professional's goals for the health visit				
Elicit the child's and family's goals and needs for the visit				
Collaborate with the family to prioritize goals for the visit				
Identify alternative ways of dealing with goals that could not be addressed during the visit				

Time Management: Session 1

CASE VIGNETTE:
JACOB'S 4 MONTH VISIT, PART 1

You arrive 30 minutes late for your clinic appointments because of the unstable condition of an infant in the NICU.

Three families are already waiting for their scheduled appointments. The first appointment is with Jacob Downing and his mother, who are here for Jacob's 4 month health visit.

When you enter the room, you notice that Jacob is fussing in his infant seat on the examining table. His mother, Eileen, is sitting on the other side of the room with a frown on her face, arms folded across her chest. This is your second health encounter with the Downing family.

Time Management: Session 1

BRIGHT FUTURES 4 MONTH VISIT: QUESTIONS FOR THE PARENT(S)

Questions for the Parent(s)

- What new things is Bobby doing?
- What questions or concerns do you have today?
- How do you know what Bobby needs or wants? Is it easy or difficult to tell?
- What have you found to be the best way to comfort him?
- How is feeding going? What do you feed Bobby?
- Tell me about Sabrina's sleeping habits. Do you put her on her back to sleep?
- Does Sabrina ride in a rear-facing infant safety seat in the back seat of the car?
- Do you think Sabrina hears all right? Sees all right?
- Do you know how to reduce the risk of lead hazards if you live in an older or recently renovated home?
- Have you returned to work or school? Do you plan to do so? What are your child care arrangements?
- Do you know what to do in case of an emergency? Do you know first aid and infant CPR?
- Is there a gun in your home? Is it unloaded and locked up? Have you considered removing the gun because of the dangers to children?

Source: Reproduced with permission from Green. M., Palfrey, J.S., Clark, E.M., & Anastasi, J.M. (Eds.) (2002). *Bright futures: Guidelines for health supervision of infants, children, and adolescents* (2nd ed., rev.)—*Pocket guide.* Arlington, VA: National Center for Education in Maternal and Child Health.

CASE VIGNETTE:
JACOB'S 4 MONTH VISIT, PART 2

Based on Eileen's responses to specific interview questions, you learn that Jacob has had intermittent and increasing fussiness for the past several weeks. He has also been waking more frequently at night.

You also learn that Eileen's mother, with whom Jacob and Eileen live, has told her daughter that Jacob has colic because she isn't taking good enough care of him.

Time Management: Session 1

FOLLOW-UP SELF-ASSESSMENT OF TIME MANAGEMENT

Time Management Self-Assessment					
Health Visit	**1**	**2**	**3**	**4**	**5**
I minimized documentation time.					
I clarified my professional goals for the health visit.					
I identified the family's and child's concerns for the visit.					
I prioritized the goals for the visit by collaborating with the family and child.					
I used alternative ways of dealing with goals that could not be addressed in the visit.					

Comments

____

____

____

Time Management: Session 1

SESSION EVALUATION FORM

Session 1: Applying the Five-Step Time Management Model

Date: _______________________________

Facilitator(s): _______________________________

Site: _______________________________

---

1. Overall, I found the "Applying the Five-Step Time Management Model" session to be:

Not Useful			Very Useful	
1	2	3	4	5

2. The objectives of the session were:

Not Clear				Clear
1	2	3	4	5

3. The organization of the session was:

Poor				Excellent
1	2	3	4	5

4. The communication skills of the facilitator(s) were:

Poor				Excellent
1	2	3	4	5

5. The facilitator(s) stimulated interest in the subject matter:

Not at All			Very Much	
1	2	3	4	5

6. The facilitator(s) encouraged group participation:

Not at All			Very Much	
1	2	3	4	5

7. Handouts or visual aids (if used) were:

Not Helpful		Very Helpful		
1	2	3	4	5

8. Any additional comments?

____

____

____

9. The most useful features of the session were:

____

____

____

10. Suggestions for improvement

____

____

____

11. Suggestions for topics related to this session

____

____

____

Time Management: Session 1

FACILITATOR SELF-ASSESSMENT FORM

Directions: Please rate yourself from 1 to 5 on the following facilitator skills. The closer you are to a 5 within each domain, the more skilled you are at facilitation. We encourage you to complete this form prior to and after each teaching experience (e.g., a single session or an entire module). This will allow you to assess your performance as a facilitator over time.

Facilitator Behavior	1	2	3	4	5
Remains neutral					
Does not judge ideas					
Keeps the group focused on common task					
Asks clarifying questions					
Creates a climate free of criticism					
Encourages participation					
Structures participation					

Source: Adapted with permission from Welch, M. (1999). *Teaching diversity and cultural competence in health care: A trainer's guide.* San Francisco, CA: Perspectives of Differences Diversity Training and Consultation for Health Professionals (PODSDT).

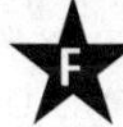

SESSION 2:

Using Encounter and Documentation Forms As Time Management Tools

At the beginning of the session, the facilitator and learners should introduce themselves briefly. (If the same group has recently completed Session 1, the facilitator may decide that introductions are not needed.) Ideas for creative introductions can be found in the Facilitator's Guide.

Setting the Context: The Bright Futures Concept

(May be omitted if recently presented or when sessions are combined.)

The facilitator (**F**) introduces the learners to the Bright Futures concept of health by reading or paraphrasing the following:

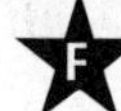

The World Health Organization has defined health as "a state of complete physical, mental and social well-being and not merely the absence of disease or infirmity." Bright Futures embraces this broad definition of health—one that includes not only prevention of morbidity and mortality, but also the achievement of a child's full potential. In the Bright Futures concept of health, providing the capacity for healthy child development is as important as ameliorating illness or injury. Recognizing and acknowledging the strengths and resources of the child, family, and community are essential to promoting healthy growth and development.

To build that capacity, the Pediatrics in Practice *curriculum focuses on six core concepts: Partnership, Communication, Health Promotion/Illness Prevention, Time Manage-ment, Education, and Advocacy. The curriculum also includes a companion module (Health) and videotape that present an overview of* Pediatrics in Practice *and the Bright Futures approach.*

Introducing the Session

Before introducing the session, the facilitator distributes the handout **Time Management: Managing Time for Health Promotion.** The facilitator may choose not to distribute the handout if it was recently given to the same learners.

Today's session is the second of two that comprise the Pediatrics in Practice *Time Manage-ment module. In the first session, we defined time management as a set of common-sense skills that help us to use time in the most effective and productive way possible. We presented a five-step model for managing time during the health visit. [Optional: Your Time Management handout outlines these steps.] The first step in that model is to maximize time for health promotion by using accurate methods that minimize documentation time.*

In today's session, our objectives will be to:

▶ *Use* Bright Futures Encounter Forms for Families *as a time management tool to identify family needs and concerns, help the family prepare for the health visit, and provide guidance on important health topics*

▶ *Become familiar with the American Academy of Pediatrics'* Well Child Visit Documentation Forms *as an effective time management tool*

▶ *Explore the use of health promotion packets in enhancing the health visit*

When we have completed the session, you should be able to answer the following questions:

▶ *How can Bright Futures and other health promotion materials help make health visits more efficient?*

> *What strategies can minimize the time spent filling out forms to document the visit?*

Discussion and Exercises

The facilitator distributes the handouts **Bright Futures Encounter Forms for Families, 4 Month Visit** and **American Academy of Pediatrics (AAP) Well Child/4 Months Visit Documentation Form.** (Both handouts include pertinent information based on the Jacob Downing case vignette discussed in Session 1.)

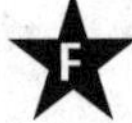 *Easy-to-use forms and educational materials are an important part of providing efficient health promotion care. Bright Futures and the American Academy of Pediatrics offer time-saving materials designed to gather and record important information for the health visit.*

These handouts provide the same kind of information that you would have at the beginning of a 4 month health visit in an office or clinic using Bright Futures Encounter Forms for Families *(available in English and in Spanish) and AAP's* Well Child Visit Documentation Forms. *Jacob's mother listed her concerns on the encounter form that she filled out in the waiting room. Professional staff have weighed and measured Jacob, taken his temperature, and recorded the information on the documentation form.*

Based on our case vignette in Session 1, you may recall that you have arrived 30 minutes late for your clinic appointments because of an infant in the NICU. Three families are already waiting for their scheduled appointments. Your first appointment is with Jacob Downing and his mother, who are here for Jacob's 4 month health visit. Take a moment to look over the information on Jacob Downing.

Reviewing the Five Steps in the Time Management Model

After allowing a few minutes for learners to familiarize themselves with the forms and review the data entered on the forms, the facilitator continues:

 *Before exploring how these forms can be used as time management tools, let's briefly review the five steps of the Time Management Model:*

> ► *Maximize time for health promotion (by minimizing documentation time)*
> ► *Clarify the health professional's goals for the visit*
> ► *Identify the family's needs and concerns*
> ► *Work with the family to prioritize goals for the visit*
> ► *Suggest other options for addressing unmet goals*

Using Encounter Forms and Other Time-Saving Techniques

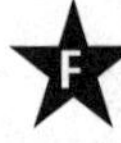 *As pediatric providers who are experiencing the pressure of time, what steps would you take to complete Jacob's visit in a timely manner?*

The learners' responses might include the following:

► Have parents complete encounter forms in the waiting room, then scan the forms before the health visit to identify any special concerns (for example, concerns about Jacob's sleep habits and colic)

► Use encounter forms for families to help explain the health visit and encourage families to identify questions or concerns they want to discuss

► Use encounter forms for families to provide anticipatory guidance on topics of special concern, such as introducing solid foods or avoiding injury by keeping one hand on the baby in high places (see "Things to Keep in Mind Between Now and the Next Visit")

► Train professional staff to help share information with the family

► Begin the physical examination while addressing some of the agenda items

► Use handouts or other patient education materials (for example, AAP's patient education handouts on sleep, feeding, other topics)

► Plan specific follow-up to address issues that could not be covered during the visit

[*Note to facilitator:* You may want to contribute your own "tried-and-true" methods, based on your professional experience.]

Using Professional Documentation Forms

After brief discussion, the facilitator continues:

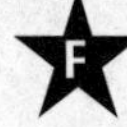 *This may be the first time that you have considered using pediatric visit documentation forms, which can minimize record-keeping time. Considering the time constraints around Jacob's visit, how can the documentation forms help accomplish the goals of the visit?*

The learners' responses might include the following:

▶ Documentation forms allow the health professional to "capture" or record all essential data and information for the visit on one page

▶ Standardized checklists for the physical exam, anticipatory guidance, and review of "systems" (feeding, sleep, behavior) require less visit preparation time and allow more time to focus on the child and family

▶ Developmental milestones and anticipatory guidance topics serve as quick-reference checkpoints for age-specific items

Putting Together Age-Specific Health Promotion Packets

After brief discussion, the facilitator continues:

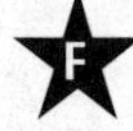 *In addition to using encounter and documentation forms, you may want to consider putting together a packet of age-specific materials that will help maximize health promotion time during the visit. Examples of these materials are listed in the Resources section of this module. For example, the Bright Futures pocket guide features effective open-ended interview questions for each recommended health visit.*

In Session 1, we used Questions for the Parent(s) to help identify goals and priorities for the 4 month visit. Bright Futures materials typically provide a menu of options. Not all items need to be covered during the visit. Using the time management steps we have discussed can help identify which items are relevant for a specific family and their health visit.

[*Note to facilitator:* Allow time for discussion.

This is an opportune time to mention patient education materials that would help the pediatric provider meet health promotion goals that might not be fully addressed because of time constraints. In addition to the Bright Futures and AAP resource materials listed under Resources at the end of the module, the use of community-based or customized patient education materials can be encouraged.]

 *Since families are also health partners, what are some ways that you could incorporate the family perspective on these packets?*

Sample responses might include:

▶ Invite one or more families to review available materials and identify which ones are most helpful

▶ Ask families what educational materials they are already using and finding helpful

▶ Pilot-test a health promotion packet you've already put together by using it during the health visit, then talking with the family about how the materials met their needs, what information (if any) was missing, and whether the materials were easy to understand

Take-Home Message

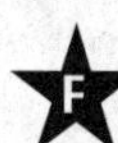 *Effective, well-designed documentation forms and encounter forms can help health professionals identify concerns quickly, minimize writing time, and adequately document the health visit. Such forms can be the basis of a health promotion packet that serves the needs of both pediatric providers and families. The reference and resource lists at the end of this module offer suggestions for both professional and family materials that might be valuable additions to your health promotion packet. Before we conclude, what questions remain about what we addressed today?*

Answers to the Guiding Questions

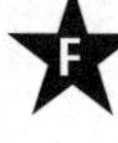 *Now that we have completed this session on Time Management, you should be able to answer the following questions:*

▶ How can Bright Futures and other health promotion materials help

make health visits more efficient?

- *Bright Futures Encounter Forms for Families*, which are available in English and in Spanish, help families prepare for the health visit, identify issues or concerns they may want to discuss with the pediatric provider, and offer guidance on health topics.

- AAP *Well Child Visit Documentation Forms* provide standard checklists for key components of the health visit and capture essential data on one page.

▶ What strategies can minimize the time spent filling out forms to document the visit?

- Ask parents to complete family encounter forms in waiting room.

- Use professional documentation forms to capture all essential data for visit.

- Use handouts or other patient education materials.

- Begin the physical examination while still addressing some of the agenda items.

- Train professional staff to help elicit and share health information with the family.

- Make plans for follow-up to address other issues.

Evaluation

The facilitator now distributes the **Session Evaluation Form**. The facilitator also completes the **Facilitator Self-Assessment Form.**

Time Management: Session 2

TIME MANAGEMENT: MANAGING TIME FOR HEALTH PROMOTION

1. Maximize time for health promotion.
- Use accurate methods that minimize documentation time
- Ask family to complete forms in waiting area
- Organize chart in consistent manner
- Scan chart before meeting with the child and family
- Train staff to elicit information and to provide follow-up with family

2. Clarify health professional's goals for visit.
- Review screening forms and other basic health data
- Observe parent-infant interaction
- Clarify key issues for visit
  Example: Review age-appropriate anticipatory guidance.
- Identify needs, then rank them in order of importance

3. Identify family's needs and concerns for visit.
- Selectively use Bright Futures general and age-appropriate interview questions
- Include open-ended questions to draw family into visit
  Example: "Tell me about Sabrina's sleeping habits. What position does she sleep in?" (Elicits more than yes/no answer, and presents "teachable moment" on "Back to Sleep" and SIDS.)

4. Work with the family to prioritize goals for visit.
- Explain purpose of visit (identify, address specific concerns and overall health and development)
- Identify family's and health professional's shared goals
- Prioritize needs through family-friendly negotiation
  Example: "I appreciate your concerns about ________. While you are here, I would also like to talk about ________."

5. Suggest other options for addressing unmet goals.
- Acknowledge importance of issues that could not be fully addressed during the visit
- Offer additional resources (handouts, audiotapes, videotapes, Web-based materials)
- Suggest a follow-up visit or phone call
  Example: "I'm sorry we weren't able to talk about ________ during today's visit. Could I call you one afternoon next week to follow up on that?"
  Or: "Would you be able to come back next week so we could talk more about that?"
- Provide referral to professional or community resource
  Example: "I know we haven't had a chance to cover your concern about ________ today. Would you like to pursue it with a specialist in that area?"

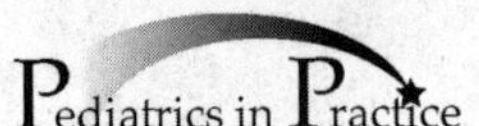

Time Management: Session 2

BRIGHT FUTURES ENCOUNTER FORMS FOR FAMILIES, 4 MONTH VISIT

4 MONTH VISIT   Date:

Name *Jacob Downing*

Age *4 months*   Weight __________   Length __________   **Bright Futures**

At Today's Visit

- You and your health professional will have an opportunity to talk about your baby's growth and development.
- Your health professional will ask for an update on your baby's health.
- Your baby will have a physical examination.
- Your baby will receive one or more immunizations: hepatitis; DTaP; Hib; polio. Ask your health professional about them.
- You will have an opportunity to ask questions.

Things You May Want to Discuss During This Visit

- How your family is getting along.
- Getting the help you need with your baby.
- How to tell what your baby wants and needs.
- Your baby's sleeping habits.
- Plans to return to work or school, and child care arrangements.
- Finding time for you and your partner to go out without your baby; choosing responsible babysitters.
- Changes in your family since your last visit.
- Some things your baby can do now that she couldn't do at the last visit.
- Any other topics you may want to discuss.

Jacob wakes a lot more at night than he used to.
What is colic? Does Jacob have colic?

Notes:

Working Together to Keep Your Child Healthy and Happy

(continued on next page)

Time Management: Session 2

BRIGHT FUTURES ENCOUNTER FORMS FOR FAMILIES, 4 MONTH VISIT (continued)

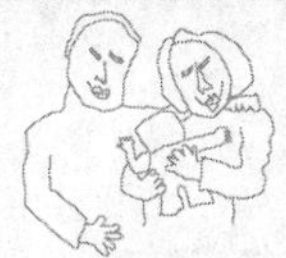

4 MONTH VISIT

Date:

Name *Jacob Downing*

Bright Futures 

Things to Keep in Mind Between Now and the Next Visit

Childproof your home. Keep medicines, cleaning aids, small or sharp objects, plastic bags, balloons, sockets, cords, and guns out of your baby's reach.

Keep the number of your local poison control center handy. Obtain a bottle of ipecac syrup but use it only when the poison control center or your health professional tells you to.

Do not put your baby in a baby walker at any age.

Always keep one hand on your baby, and do not leave him alone in the bathtub or on high places.

Introduce solid foods gradually (one per week). Start with iron-fortified baby cereal, then pureed foods (fruits or vegetables, then meats).

Do not put your baby to bed with a bottle or prop it in her mouth.

Establish a bedtime routine, and put your baby to bed while he's awake.

Encourage your partner and other children to help out with the baby.

How to Prepare for the Next Visit

Share with family members and other caregivers what you've learned at today's visit.

Keep track of illnesses and injuries including visits to other health facilities and the emergency room.

Be prepared to share information about your baby's possible allergies to food or medication.

Talk with family members and your baby's other caregivers about issues they might want you to raise with the health professional.

Keep a list of topics you would like to discuss at your next visit.

What to Expect at the Next Visit

Your baby will have a physical examination.

Your baby will receive one or more immunizations.

Notes:

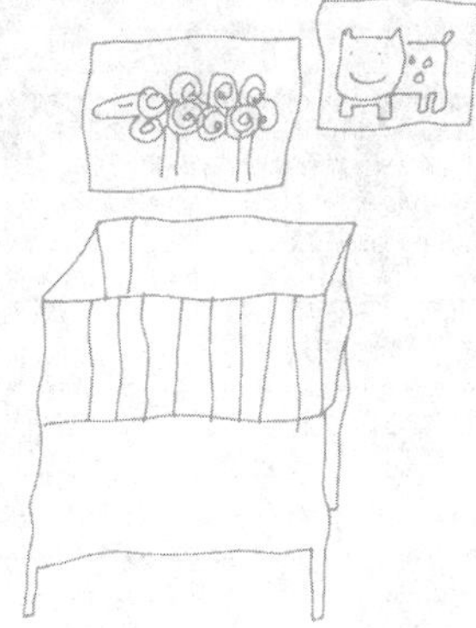

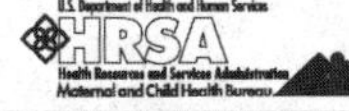

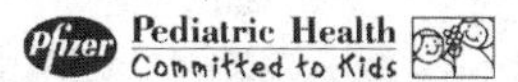

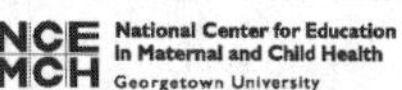

Source: Reproduced with permission from National Center for Education in Maternal and Child Health. 2002. *Bright futures: Guidelines for health supervision of infants, children, and adolescents—Encounter forms for families* (2nd ed.). Arlington, VA: National Center for Education in Maternal and Child Health.

Time Management: Session 2

AMERICAN ACADEMY OF PEDIATRICS WELL CHILD/4 MONTHS VISIT DOCUMENTATION FORM

ACCOMPANIED BY	DATE/TIME	Name
Eileen Downing, mother		Jacob Downing

DRUG ALLERGIES	CURRENT MEDICATIONS	ID NUMBER

WEIGHT (%)	HEIGHT (%)	HEAD CIRC (%)	TEMPERATURE	BIRTH DATE	AGE
5.4 Kg (10th%) See growth chart.	59 cm (5th%)	42 cm	99.4		4 months Ⓜ F

History

Concerns and questions __________________

____

____

____

Follow-up on previous concerns __________________

____

Interval history   1 None   __________________

____

Social/Family History

See Initial History Questionnaire.   1 No interval change __________

Family situation   1 No interval change __________

Parents working outside home: 1 Mother   1 Father

Child care: 1 Yes   1 No   Type __________

Changes since last visit __________________

Review of Systems

See Initial History Questionnaire and Problem List.

1 No interval change

Changes since last visit __________________

____

Nutrition: 1 Breast   1 Bottle

Formula __________ Ounces/day __________

Solid foods __________________

____

Source of water __________ Vitamins __________

Elimination: 1 NL __________________

Sleep: 1 NL __________________

Behavior: 1 NL __________________

Toxic exposure: Passive smoking   1 Yes   1 No

Development

1GROSS MOTOR	1FINE MOTOR	1COMMUNICATION
1Holds head erect	1Reaches for and	1Coos
1Raises body on hands with head up	grabs objects	1Blows bubbles, makes "raspberry sounds"
1Rolls front to back	1Brings hands together	
	1SENSORY	1SOCIAL
	1Responds to sounds	1Social smile
	1Follows objects	1Laughs or squeals

American Academy of Pediatrics

DEDICATED TO THE HEALTH OF ALL CHILDREN®

Physical Examination

"= NL

1GENERAL APPEARANCE	1LUNGS	1EXTREMITIES/HIPS
1HEAD/FONTANELLE	1HEART	1BACK
1EYES/RED REFLEX/STRABISMUS/ APPEARS TO SEE	1FEMORAL PULSES	1SKIN
1EARS/APPEARS TO HEAR	1ABDOMEN	1NEUROLOGIC
1NOSE	1GENITALIA	
1MOUTH AND THROAT	1MALE/TESTES DOWN	
	1FEMALE	

Abnormal findings and comments __________________

____

____

____

____

Assessment

1 Well child

____

____

____

Anticipatory Guidance

Discussed and/or handout given

1NUTRITION	1ELIMINATION	1INJURY PREVENTION
1Milk	1SLEEP	1Auto/Car seat
1Breastfeeding	1BEHAVIOR AND DEVELOPMENT	1Burns
1Formula (supplement or if not breastfed)	1Social	1Smoke detectors
1Solid foods	1Communication skills	1Falls
1When and how to add	1Physical	1Choking
1No honey		1Sun
		1Guns

Plan

Immunizations (See Vaccine Administration Record.)

Laboratory results __________________

____

____

Follow-up/Next visit __________________

____

____

Print Name	Signature
NURSE	
PHYSICIAN	

WELL CHILD/4 months

Time Management: Session 2

SESSION EVALUATION FORM

Session 2: Using Encounter and Documentation Forms As Time Management Tools

Date: _______________________________

Facilitator(s): _______________________________

Site: _______________________________

1. Overall, I found the "Using Encounter and Documentation Forms As Time Management Tools" session to be:

Not Useful			Very Useful	
1	2	3	4	5

2. The objectives of the session were:

Not Clear				Clear
1	2	3	4	5

3. The organization of the session was:

Poor				Excellent
1	2	3	4	5

4. The communication skills of the facilitator(s) were:

Poor				Excellent
1	2	3	4	5

5. The facilitator(s) stimulated interest in the subject matter:

Not at All			Very Much	
1	2	3	4	5

6. The facilitator(s) encouraged group participation:

Not at All			Very Much	
1	2	3	4	5

7. Handouts or visual aids (if used) were:

Not Helpful		Very Helpful		
1	2	3	4	5

8. Any additional comments?

____

____

____

9. The most useful features of the session were:

____

____

____

10. Suggestions for improvement

____

____

____

11. Suggestions for topics related to this session

____

____

____

Time Management: Session 2

FACILITATOR SELF-ASSESSMENT FORM

Directions: Please rate yourself from 1 to 5 on the following facilitator skills. The closer you are to a 5 within each domain, the more skilled you are at facilitation. We encourage you to complete this form prior to and after each teaching experience (e.g., a single session or an entire module). This will allow you to assess your performance as a facilitator over time.

Facilitator Behavior	1	2	3	4	5
Remains neutral					
Does not judge ideas					
Keeps the group focused on common task					
Asks clarifying questions					
Creates a climate free of criticism					
Encourages participation					
Structures participation					

Source: Adapted with permission from Welch, M. (1999). *Teaching diversity and cultural competence in health care: A trainer's guide.* San Francisco, CA: Perspectives of Differences Diversity Training and Consultation for Health Professionals (PODSDT).

References

American Academy of Pediatrics. (2002). *Well child/4 months visit documentation form.* Elk Grove Village, IL: American Academy of Pediatrics.

American Academy of Pediatrics. (2004). *Periodic Survey of Fellows,* 56. Elk Grove Village, IL: American Academy of Pediatrics.

Bartlett, E.E. (1999). Always running behind? Try these time-management tips. *Medical Economics, 76*(4), 83, 86, 91.

Benjamin, J.T., Cimino, S.A., Hafler, J.P., Bright Futures Health Promotion Work Group, & Bernstein, H.H. (2002). The office visit: A time to promote health—but how? *Contemporary Pediatrics, 19*(2), 90–107.

Bonfield, A., [prod.] (2000). *Bright futures: Health supervision of infants, children, and adolescents* [videotape, part of the Pediatrics in Practice health promotion curriculum]. Sharon, MA: Biomedical Video and Multimedia.

Forsch, R.T. (2003), Improving office operations. *Clinics in Family Practice, 5*(4), 1009.

Glascoe, F.P., Oberkalid, F., Dworkin, P.H., & Trimm, F. (1998). Brief approaches to educating patients and parents in primary care. *Pediatrics, 101*(6), E10.

Green, M., & Palfrey, J.S., (Eds.) (2002). *Bright futures: Guidelines for health supervision of infants, children, and adolescents* (2nd ed., rev.). Arlington, VA: National Center for Education in Maternal and Child Health.

Green, M., Palfrey, J.S., Clark, E.M., & Anastasi, J.M., (Eds.) (2002). *Bright futures: Guidelines for health supervision of infants, children, and adolescents* (2nd ed., rev.)—*Pocket guide.* Arlington, VA: National Center for Education in Maternal and Child Health.

Maher, C.A. (1982). Time management training for providers of special services. *Exceptional Children, 48*(6), 523–528.

National Center for Education in Maternal and Child Health. (2002). *Bright futures: Guidelines for health supervision of infants, children, and adolescents—Encounter forms for families* (2nd ed.). Arlington, VA: National Center for Education in Maternal and Child Health.

Schor, E.L. (2004), Rethinking well-child care. *Pediatrics, 114*(1), 210-216.

Schroeder, R.E. (1998). Using time management to achieve balance. *Medical Group Management Journal, 45*(6), 20–26, 28.

Resources

American Academy of Pediatrics (Selected Materials)
Descriptions of materials and ordering information available online at www.aap.org.

American Academy of Pediatrics. (1997). *Guidelines for health supervision III.* Elk Grove Village, IL: American Academy of Pediatrics.

American Academy of Pediatrics. (1994). *The injury prevention program (TIPP).* Elk Grove Village, IL: American Academy of Pediatrics.

American Academy of Pediatrics. (2000). *Patient education on CD-ROM* (2nd ed.). Elk Grove Village, IL: American Academy of Pediatrics.

Bright Futures (Selected Materials)
Descriptions of materials and ordering information available online at www.brightfutures.org. Many materials can be viewed online and downloaded.

Jellinek, M., Patel, B.P., & Froehle, M.C., (Eds.) (2002). *Bright futures in practice: Mental health* (2 vols.). Arlington, VA: National Center for Education in Maternal and Child Health.

National Center for Education in Maternal and Child Health. (2002). *Bright futures child health record: From birth through 6 years of age* [English or Spanish]. Arlington, VA: National Center for Education in Maternal and Child Health.

National Center for Education in Maternal and Child Health. (2002). *Bright futures nutrition family fact sheets* [English or Spanish]. Arlington, VA: National Center for Education in Maternal and Child Health.

National Center for Education in Maternal and Child Health. (2001). *Bright futures family tip sheets.* Arlington, VA: National Center for Education in Maternal and Child Health.

National Center for Education in Maternal and Child Health. (1996). *Bright futures: Guidelines for health supervision of infants, children, and adolescents—Anticipatory guidance cards.* Arlington, VA: National Center for Education in Maternal and Child Health.

Patrick, K., Spear, B., Holt, K., & Sofka, D. (2001). *Bright futures in Practice: physical activity.* Arlington, VA: National Center for Education in Maternal and Child Health.

Story, M., Holt, K., Sofka, D., & Clark, E.M. (2002). *Bright futures in practice: Nutrition—Pocket guide.* Arlington, VA: National Center for Education in Maternal and Child Health.

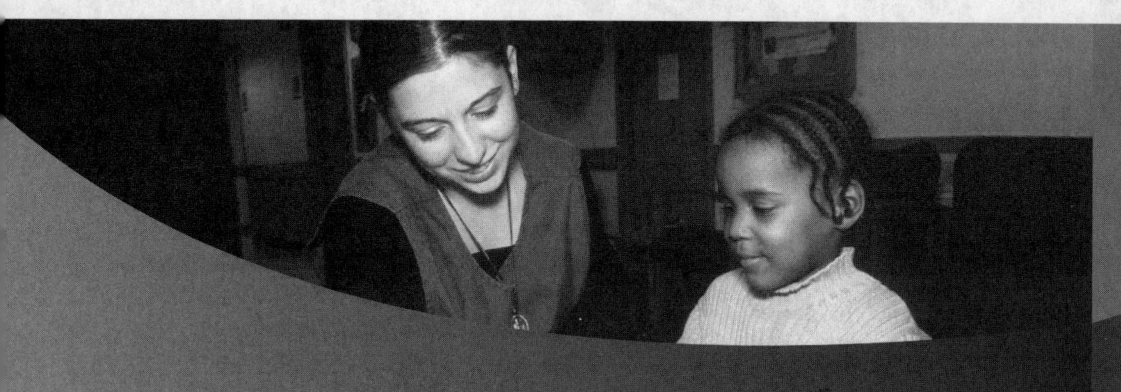

Chapter 7

Education

Educating Families Through Teachable Moments

Donna M. D'Alessandro

Judith S. Palfrey

Janet P. Hafler

CONTENTS

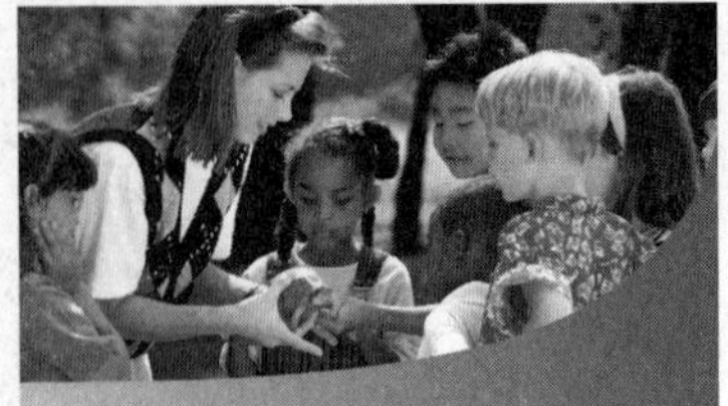

EDUCATION
Educating Families Through Teachable Moments

OVERVIEW

Background

Opportunities to promote learning occur many times a day but often go unrecognized. Identifying daily teaching "moments" and knowing how to improve the health education of children, families, and communities is critical to fostering health promotion. Teachable moments can occur any time that children and families are ready to learn, and the health visit presents the ideal opportunity for the child health professional to teach. The child health professional must not only recognize teachable moments but also respond to them by using suitable and effective teaching strategies.

Goal

The overall goal of this module is to improve the health education of children, families, and communities by introducing the Teachable Moments model and by identifying teaching strategies that address daily teaching opportunities.

This module will enable learners to:

▶ Recognize the teachable moment
▶ Use a variety of teaching strategies
▶ Facilitate learning with children and families

Instructional Design

This module consists of two 30-minute sessions:

▶ Session 1 introduces the Teachable Moments model and offers a variety of teaching strategies that may be used to facilitate learning.
▶ Session 2 elaborates on the Teachable Moments model and further explores communication skills.

▶ Each of the two sessions can be used as a separate, stand-alone offering, or the sessions can be combined. See the Facilitator's Guide for information on combining sessions.
▶ If Session 1 is not presented, the early part of Session 2 (a recap of information from Session 1) should be expanded somewhat in its explanation of Teachable Moments.

Teaching Strategies

The teaching strategies used in this module include mini-presentation, case discussion, role-play, and reflective exercise. These strategies have been selected to help learners develop the skills required to recognize teachable moments and facilitate learning with children and families. Please refer to the Facilitator's Guide for more information related to each strategy.

Evaluation

Learners will complete a **Session Evaluation Form** following each session. Learners will also be given a **Preceptor Structured Observation Form** and a **Patient and Family Survey Form** for use in their practice settings. Facilitators are encouraged to complete a **Facilitator Self-Assessment Form** prior to and following each teaching experience (e.g., a single session or an entire module) in order to assess their own performance over time.

Guiding Questions

Learners who have completed the entire Education module should be able to answer the following questions:

▶ How do I identify teaching opportunities during my health encounters with children and families?

- ► How do I partner with the child and family to begin teaching?
- ► How do I decide which teaching strategy (strategies) to use?

INTRODUCTION TO TEACHING SESSIONS

Session 1: Teachable Moments

Objectives

The objectives for this session are for the facilitator to:

- ► Introduce the Teachable Moments model
- ► Offer a variety of teaching strategies that may be used to facilitate learning
- ► Present the advantages, disadvantages, and appropriate use of specific teaching strategies

Materials

The materials and teaching aids needed for this session are:

Handouts

- ► Education: Educating Families Through Teachable Moments
- ► Case Vignette: The Thermometer
- ► Alternate Case Vignette: The Inhaler
- ► Chart of Teaching Strategies
- ► Session Evaluation Form
- ► Preceptor Structured Observation Form
- ► Patient and Family Survey Form

Facilitator Form

- ► Facilitator Self-Assessment Form

Teaching Aids

- ► Display board, flip chart, or chalkboard
- ► Markers or chalk
- ► Paper and pens or pencils
- ► Glass thermometer, coffee stirrer, or paper equivalent
- ► Demonstration metered-dose inhaler or paper equivalent (if the alternate case vignette is used)

- ► Patient education materials (written and/or demonstration models) on how to take a temperature or use a metered-dose inhaler (optional)

Time

The time allocated for this session is 30 minutes.

Session 2: Making the Most of Teachable Moments

Objectives

The objectives for this session are for the facilitator to:

- ► Provide an in-depth look at the Teachable Moments model
- ► Explore communication skills such as the use of questions and wait time as they apply to the Teachable Moment

Materials

The materials and teaching aids needed for this session are:

Handouts

- ► Education: Educating Families Through Teachable Moments
- ► Case Vignette: The Polio Shot
- ► Questioning and Nonquestioning Techniques
- ► Session Evaluation Form
- ► Preceptor Structured Observation Form
- ► Patient and Family Survey Form

Facilitator Form

- ► Facilitator Self-Assessment Form

Teaching Aids

- ► Overhead projector
- ► Overhead of the Education: Educating Families Through Teachable Moments handout (optional)
- ► Overhead of Questioning Exercise

Time

The time allocated for this session is 30 minutes.

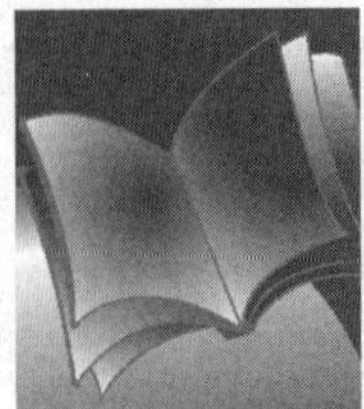

SESSION 1:
Teachable Moments

At the beginning of the session, the facilitator and learners should introduce themselves briefly. Ideas for creative introductions can be found in the Facilitator's Guide.

Setting the Context: The Bright Futures Concept

The facilitator **(F)** introduces the learners to the Bright Futures concept of health by reading or paraphrasing the following:

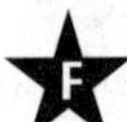
The World Health Organization has defined health as "a state of complete physical, mental and social well-being and not merely the absence of disease or infirmity." Bright Futures embraces this broad definition of health—one that includes not only prevention of morbidity and mortality, but also the achievement of a child's full potential. In the Bright Futures concept of health, providing the capacity for healthy child development is as important as ameliorating illness or injury. Recognizing and acknowledging the strengths and resources of the child, family, and community are essential to promoting healthy growth and development.

To build that capacity, the Pediatrics in Practice curriculum focuses on six core concepts: Partnership, Communication, Health Promotion/ Illness Prevention, Time Management, Education, and Advocacy. The curriculum also includes a companion module (Health) and videotape that present an overview of Pediatrics in Practice and the Bright Futures approach.

Introducing the Session

Before introducing the session, the facilitator distributes the handout **Education: Educating Families Through Teachable Moments** to the learners.

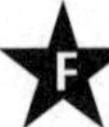
Today's session is the first of two that comprise the Pediatrics in Practice Education module. We are going to explore a teaching model you can use with the children and families you encounter each day. The model is based on a concept called Teachable Moments.

Opportunities to promote learning occur many times a day but often go unrecognized. Identifying daily teachable moments and knowing how to improve the health education of children, families, and communities is critical to fostering health promotion. Teachable moments can occur any time that children and families are ready to learn, and the health visit presents the ideal opportunity for the child health professional to teach. The pediatric provider must not only recognize teachable moments but also respond to them by using suitable and effective teaching strategies.

In today's session, our objectives will be to:
- ▶ *Define teachable moments*
- ▶ *Identify the six steps in the Teachable Moments model*
- ▶ *Describe a variety of teaching strategies*
- ▶ *Apply the six-step teaching model to a case vignette*
- ▶ *Practice using teaching strategies based on the case vignette*

When we have completed the session, you should be able to answer the following question:
- ▶ *How do I identify teaching opportunities during my health encounters with children and families?*

The facilitator asks the learners to look at the **Education: Educating Families Through Teachable Moments** handout.

Let's begin by taking a look at the definition of a teachable moment. Next, we will identify the six steps of the Teachable Moments model.

Discussion and Exercises

Defining a Teachable Moment

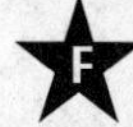 *A teachable moment is simply any time during the course of a health visit when the child health professional identifies an opportunity to teach the child and family. Teachable moments are the moments when the child and family are ready to learn.*

After the definition has been read, the facilitator continues:

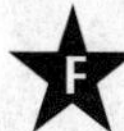 *These teachable moments occur many times each day but often go unrecognized.*

The Six-Step Teachable Moments Model

 *There are six important steps in the Teachable Moments model. These steps will help us take advantage of those teaching opportunities that are sometimes missed.*

> **1. Recognize teachable moments in the health visit**
>
> *The child or the family will often express a need to learn during the health visit.*
>
> **2. Clarify the learning needs of the child and family**
>
> *Assess and clarify the family's learning needs. Determine what the family knows and needs to know.*
>
> **3. Set a limited agenda and prioritize needs together**
>
> *Plan for the appropriate teaching strategy by setting a limited agenda and prioritizing the learning needs together with the family.*
>
> **4. Select a teaching strategy**
>
> *Select and implement the appropriate teaching strategy or combination of strategies.*
>
> **5. Seek and provide feedback**
>
> *Seek and provide feedback about the information you've presented. Did the family understand? Can they affirm the knowledge you've provided? Were there any misunderstandings that need to be corrected?*
>
> **6. Evaluate the effectiveness of the teaching**
>
> *Obtain the family's perspective on the teaching you've provided. Will they remember the infor-mation after they leave the visit? If learning a new skill was involved, were they able to demonstrate the skill for you?*

The facilitator next offers the four characteristics of the teachable moment.

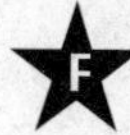 *Now, let's look at the four characteristics of the teachable moment.*

The teachable moment:

> ▶ *Provides "information bites" or small amounts of information*
>
> ▶ *Is directed at the child's or family's specific need*
>
> ▶ *Is brief, requiring only a few seconds of time*
>
> ▶ *Requires no preparation time*

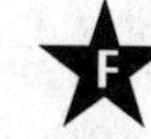 *Do you have any questions about the Teach-able Moments model?*

Case Vignette: The Thermometer

After discussing the Teachable Moments model, the facilitator distributes copies of the case vignette handout **The Thermometer.**

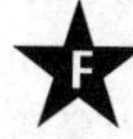 *We'll use this case vignette as we apply the six steps of the Teachable Moments model. Would someone like to read the vignette for us?*

Alternate Case Vignette: The Inhaler

The facilitator may choose to present the alternate case vignette. This vignette can be used instead of the thermometer case vignette, using the same questions when applying the six steps of the Teachable Moments model and the same instructions for the group exercise. In the group exercise, the "showing" (demonstration) group may use a demonstration metered-dose inhaler or a rolled and folded piece of paper.

Applying the Six Steps

Using the display board, the facilitator asks learners to suggest responses to each of the six steps below. The facilitator may use the examples that are provided, if needed.

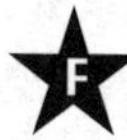 *The focus of this discussion is the implementa-tion of each step of the model. Please suggest elements of the case vignette that illustrate each of the six steps as we go through the list.*

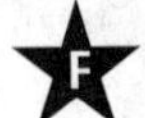

1. **Recognize teachable moments in the health visit**

   ▶ Mei and Li are not sure how to use the thermometer properly

2. **Clarify the learning needs of the child and family**

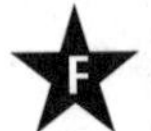

   What is it they need to learn?

   ▶ The mechanics of using a thermometer

   ▶ When to take a temperature

   ▶ What the readings mean

   ▶ When to call for help based on the readings

3. **Set a limited agenda and prioritize needs together**

   What information does the family want?

   ▶ They need help with all of the topics (above)

   ▶ They want to learn how to use and read the thermometer now

   ▶ They are worried they will not remember what the readings mean

4. **Select a teaching strategy**

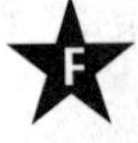

   From the list of six teaching strategies noted in the model, which strategies could apply in this case?

   ▶ Telling—explaining and giving directions on the use of the thermometer

   ▶ Showing—demonstrating the use of the thermometer

   ▶ Providing resources—giving the family an information sheet on the use of the thermometer

5. **Seek and provide feedback**

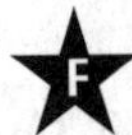

   For the method(s) you selected (telling, showing, providing resources), how might you receive feedback?

   ▶ Mei and Li thank you and tell you that they understand how and when to use the thermometer

6. **Evaluate the effectiveness of the teaching**

   How would you assess whether the teaching was helpful and effective?

   ▶ Ask Mei and Li to practice in front of you and demonstrate the proper use of the thermometer

Group Exercise

The facilitator divides the learners into three teaching teams and assigns each of them one of the teaching strategies. (With a smaller group of learners, use two teams; with a larger group, include as many strategies and teams as needed.)

The teaching teams are assigned a task appropriate to each of the teaching strategies.

For example:

Teaching Team A will use the "telling" strategy and will provide Mei and Li with a 1-minute explanation on the use of a thermometer.

This team will need paper and pens. Instruct learners to write down each step in the order that it will be presented and to pay close attention to the exact wording of the explanation.

Teaching Team B will use the "showing" strategy and will develop and provide Mei and Li with a 1-minute demonstration on how to use a thermometer.

This team will need a glass thermometer, a coffee stirrer, or a rolled piece of paper.

Teaching Team C will use the strategy of "providing resources" and will design a one-page patient information handout on how to use a thermometer and will show it to Mei and Li.

This team will need paper for writing.

Encourage learners to think about different elements to include in the handout, including how the information should be worded and what illustrations might be appropriate.

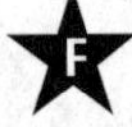

Imagine that you are Mei or Li and ask yourself what you would want and need to know. Be very explicit with the details you provide as you teach.

Each team has 5 minutes to work together on its assigned task. One person from each team will then act as the "teacher" for the other teams of learners who will assume the roles of Mei and Li. The "teacher" must use only the teaching strategy his or her group worked on. Imagine that your strategy will be the only way Mei and Li will receive the information.

Evaluating the Teaching Strategies

Each group presents its finished product. After each presentation, the facilitator asks all learners the following questions, recording the responses on the display board.

Pediatrics in Practice

 ▶ *Was this teaching strategy effective in teaching Mei and Li how to use a thermometer?*

▶ *Why or why not?*

▶ *What could be improved?*

▶ *Under what circumstances would the strategy have been successful? What circumstances would make it a less effective one?*

The facilitator should outline the following points if they have not been made during the presentations.

 ▶ *Teaching strategies are often used in combination. For example, you might provide the child and family with information verbally and also give them a handout to take home after the visit.*

▶ *Combining strategies helps families remember the information better. They can "experience" the learning in more than just one way.*

▶ *Different strategies used together help accommodate the family's different learning styles.*

▶ *Some teaching strategies are reinforcing and enduring. Handouts provide the opportunity for the family to look at the information from a different perspective and to refer to the material again later.*

▶ *Another reinforcing and enduring option is to give an "information prescription" for families. Families can then find additional resources for themselves (e.g., books, videos, or Web sites).*

The facilitator might then ask each teaching team to brainstorm about the relative advantages and disadvantages of their respective approaches. The facilitator and the learners can build a chart (similar to the one above) using these and other points that are raised.

The facilitator may use some of the following questions to build and elaborate on the key learning points of the exercise.

 • *What were some problems the teams encountered in developing or presenting their strategies?*

• *How did you decide which teaching strategy (strategies) to use?*

• *What combination of strategies would have ensured that Mei and Li learned what they needed to know?*

Take-Home Message

The facilitator summarizes the session:

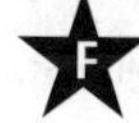 *During this session, we've discussed recognizing teachable moments and using effective*

TEACHING STRATEGY	Advantages	Disadvantages
Telling	• Can provide families with information. • Can make the same point many times. • Can clarify concepts.	• Learners may be confused and not say so. • May be hard to remember all of the information. • There is nothing for the family to take home.
Showing	• Provides a step-by-step demonstration. • Provider can talk and model at the same time.	• May take time and equipment to set up. • There may be nothing for the family to take home.
Providing Resources	• Can explain the information. • May have pictures to illustrate concepts. • Is something to take home.	• May not convey all (or may convey too much) of the information. • Families may not be able to read it. It may get lost.

teaching strategies after the teachable moment has been identified. We have also seen that each teaching strategy has strengths and weaknesses and that combining teaching strategies often works best. Before we conclude, what questions remain about what we addressed today?

The facilitator distributes the **Chart of Teaching Strategies** handout and says:

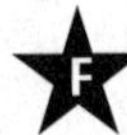 *This handout summarizes various teaching strategies, their advantages and disadvantages, and examples of situations where they might be effective. Although not all of these strategies would be appropriate to use with families, you may find yourself in other situations where this information would be helpful. It is a more comprehensive reference on teaching strategies than what we have presented today. Please take some time to review the chart. We can take time during clinic today or at another time to go over any questions you may have.*

Answer to the Guiding Question

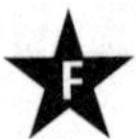 *Now that we have completed this session on Education, you should be able to answer the following question:*

- How do I identify teaching opportunities during my health encounters with children and families?
  - Learn to recognize teachable moments during the course of a health visit
  - Focus on the family and listen actively to what they ask or say
  - Look for moments to teach when the child and family are ready to learn

Planning for the Next Session (if Session 2 is planned)

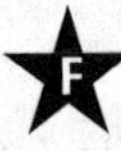 *In the next session, we will take an in-depth look at the Teachable Moments model and explore the use of questions and wait time as they apply to the Teachable Moment.*

The facilitator asks the learners to prepare for the next session by considering the following:

- How do I partner with the child and family to begin teaching?

- How do I decide which teaching strategy (strategies) to use?

Optional Follow-up Exercises

If Session 2 of the Education module is planned, the facilitator may choose to assign one of the exercises presented below.

If Session 2 is not planned, the facilitator might consider assigning one of these optional exercises and following up with the learners at a future time. One of the exercises could also be assigned as a self-motivating exercise for the learners.

Observation of Teachable Moments

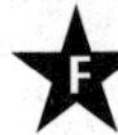 *In your health visits today and over the next week, practice identifying the teachable moments you experience, either as a teacher yourself or as an observer of another person teaching.*

Keep a list (in a journal or on 3" x 5" cards) and briefly make notes about the teachable moments as they occur. Also note the teaching strategy (or strategies) you or the other person used in response to the teachable moment. Make notes right away or as soon as possible later in the day.

Use of Teaching Strategies

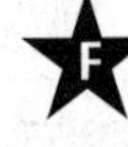 *During the next week, set a goal to use at least one teaching strategy you would not normally use during your health visits with children and families. Make notes about the strategies you used and how effective you think they were.*

Review and Critique of Patient Education Materials

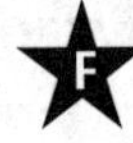 *Review and critique patient education materials on taking temperatures (or using a metered-dose inhaler). Practice using various types of thermometers (or equipment such as spacers).*

Evaluation

The facilitator now distributes the **Session Evaluation Form**, the **Preceptor Structured Observation Form**, and the **Patient and Family Survey Form**. The facilitator also completes the **Facilitator Self-Assessment Form**.

Education: Session 1

EDUCATION: EDUCATING FAMILIES THROUGH TEACHABLE MOMENTS

A teachable moment is simply any time during the course of a health visit when the child health professional identifies an opportunity to teach the child and family. Teachable moments are the moments when the child and family are ready to learn.

1. Recognize "teachable moments" in health visit

2. Clarify learning needs of child and family

3. Set a limited agenda and prioritize needs together

4. Select teaching strategy

5. Seek and provide feedback

6. Evaluate effectiveness of teaching

Four characteristics of the teachable moment

- Provides "information bites" (small amounts of information)
- Is directed to the child's or family's specific need
- Is brief (e.g., a few seconds)
- Requires no preparation time

Teaching Strategies	Advantages
Telling (explain, provide information, give directions)	Works well when giving initial explanations or clarifying concepts
Showing (demonstrate, model, draw)	Illustrates concepts for visual learners
Providing resources (handouts, videos, Web sites)	Serves as reference after family leaves the office/clinic
Questioning (ask open-ended questions, allow time for response)	Promotes problem-solving, critical thinking; elicits better information; stimulates recall
Practicing (apply new information)	Reinforces new concepts
Giving constructive feedback (seek family's perspective, correct misunderstandings, restate, clarify)	Affirms family's knowledge; corrects misunderstandings

Source: Reproduced with permission from Green. M., Palfrey, J.S., Clark, E.M., & Anastasi, J.M. (Eds.) (2002). *Bright futures: Guidelines for health supervision of infants, children, and adolescents* (2nd ed., rev.)—*Pocket guide.* Arlington, VA: National Center for Education in Maternal and Child Health.

Education: Session 1

CASE VIGNETTE:
THE THERMOMETER

Mei and Li are first-time parents of a 1-week-old son in your clinic. You have 5 more minutes to spend with them in the visit. After you discuss the baby's temperature, Mei and Li tell you that they were given a glass thermometer as a baby gift. They inform you that they don't know how to use the thermometer.

Education: Session 1

CASE VIGNETTE:
THE INHALER

Amanda is an 8-year-old girl who comes to see you with her parents. Recently, her asthma flare-ups have been getting worse. In the past, Amanda needed intermittent treatment of her asthma. Amanda, her parents, and you decide together to begin daily anti-inflammatory treatment using an inhaler and spacer.

Education: Session 1

CHART OF TEACHING STRATEGIES

STRATEGY	Advantages	Disadvantages	Example Situation
Apprenticeship/ Preceptorship	Begins to change behavior with personalized instruction.	Very time and resource intensive.	Continuity clinic, a day spent with a lobbyist.
Brainstorming	Good for generating initial ideas, learning others' points of view.	Needs several people and some setup and recording. Ideas need to be further developed.	Discussion of possible solutions for staffing. Discussion of different community-based options for care and pros/cons.
Computer-Assisted Instruction	Good for initial instruction, practice, repetitions, and future reference.	Learner may need to obtain basic computer skills before using, may have "mechanical" quality.	Anticipatory guidance on development, safety, community activities.
Demonstration/ Modeling	Illustrates concepts for visual learners.	May take time and equipment to set up.	How to perform age-appropriate developmental assessment. How to wear a bicycle helmet properly.
Discussion	Good for problem-solving, critical thinking, demonstrating different points of view.	May take time for the concepts to evolve, some in group may not participate.	Discussion of community approaches to child health problems. Discussion of strategies that different learners have found effective.
Feedback	Affirms knowledge, corrects misunderstandings, begins to change behavior, essential for learning.	The teacher may not give useful feedback or may not give any feedback at all.	Asking a supervisor how your procedures or techniques could improve. Asking a patient or family member how helpful suggestions for behavior change have been.
Handouts/Printed Materials	Often used to illustrate initially; useful for later reference.	Information may not convey nuances, quantity of information may overwhelm.	Handouts on discipline that works, TV charts for logging hours watched.
Lectures	Works well for initial explanation or clarifying concepts.	Teacher centered, not learner centered. Generally cannot review the presentation.	Review of the biochemical actions of new vaccines, normal cardiac electrophysiology, or medical treatment plan.

(continued on next page)

Education: Session 1

CHART OF TEACHING STRATEGIES (continued)

STRATEGY	Advantages	Disadvantages	Example Situation
Practicing	Begins to change behavior with personalized instruction, reinforces concepts.	Takes time, may need observation from an instructor.	Practicing new ways of eliciting history. Going over new methods of performing pubertal exam, using asthma inhaler properly.
Problem-Solving	Provides opportunity to apply critical thinking skills. Also see Practicing.	Takes time and requires commitment and mastery.	Working with parent on child care options, advocating for window guards in housing complex.
Questioning	Promotes problem-solving, critical thinking; elicits better information; stimulates recall.	Can be too teacher centered.	What is the patient's/family members' knowledge of nutritional needs? What feeding techniques has the family learned?
Reading	Good for instruction, future reference, further exploration.	No interaction with people.	Update on attention deficit hyperactivity disorder (ADHD); what constipation is and how it can be managed.
Review/ Repetition	Reinforces concepts learned.	Takes time.	How are tooth-brushing, flossing being carried out? No guns in the home.
Role-Playing	Good in helping learner apply material.	Learners may feel threatened; it may be difficult to relate to the character or situation.	Giving feedback to a junior learner, supporting patient/family members in making plans or decisions.
Slides	Similar to lectures.	Information is very brief, cannot easily repeat the information.	Reinforce specific verbal points such as immunization schedule.
Videotapes	Good in support of content in a lecture.	Need audiovisual equipment, may be difficult to relate to the character or situation.	Wide range of child health topics, particularly effective for demonstrating group approaches.

Education: Session 1

SESSION EVALUATION FORM

Session 1: Teachable Moments

Date: _______________________________

Facilitator(s): _______________________________________

Site: _______________________________________

---

1. Overall, I found the "Teachable Moments" session to be:

Not Useful			Very Useful	
1	2	3	4	5

2. The objectives of the session were:

Not Clear				Clear
1	2	3	4	5

3. The organization of the session was:

Poor				Excellent
1	2	3	4	5

4. The communication skills of the facilitator(s) were:

Poor				Excellent
1	2	3	4	5

5. The facilitator(s) stimulated interest in the subject matter:

Not at All			Very Much	
1	2	3	4	5

6. The facilitator(s) encouraged group participation:

Not at All			Very Much	
1	2	3	4	5

7. Handouts or visual aids (if used) were:

Not Helpful		Very Helpful		
1	2	3	4	5

8. Any additional comments?

   ____
   ____
   ____

9. The most useful features of the session were:

   ____
   ____
   ____

10. Suggestions for improvement

   ____
   ____
   ____

11. Suggestions for topics related to this session

   ____
   ____
   ____

Education: Session 1

PRECEPTOR STRUCTURED OBSERVATION FORM

Effective Behaviors Using the Teachable Moments Model			
Behavior	*Observed*	*Not Observed*	*Not Applicable*
Recognizes "teachable moments" in the health visit			
Clarifies the learning needs of the child and family			
Sets a limited agenda and prioritizes learning needs with the child and family			
Selects appropriate teaching strategy			
Uses teaching materials appropriately (e.g., handouts)			
Seeks feedback from and provides feedback to the child and family			
Evaluates effectiveness of teaching			
Uses teaching time appropriately during the health visit			

Comments

____

____

____

____

____

____

____

____

Education: Session 1

PATIENT AND FAMILY SURVEY FORM

To our Patients and Families:

The child health professionals in our clinic are very interested in your opinions about the care that we provide for you and your child. As part of our effort to continue to improve the care we offer, we ask that you please complete this survey about today's visit. Your responses will be confidential and will not be shared directly with your child health professional.

Thank you for your time in completing this survey.

The Staff of the Clinic

PATIENT AND FAMILY SURVEY	I am a: ☐ Patient ☐ Family Member				
My Child Health Professional:	**Disagree <—> Uncertain <—> Agree**				
Recognized that I wanted to learn more about an issue	1	2	3	4	5
Helped me to make clear what I wanted to learn	1	2	3	4	5
Helped me to talk about the most important issues first	1	2	3	4	5
Gave me the information clearly so I could understand it	1	2	3	4	5
Asked me what I did or did not understand	1	2	3	4	5
Gave me enough time to talk about my concerns	1	2	3	4	5

Comments

____

____

____

____

____

____

____

____

____

____

Education: Session 1

FACILITATOR SELF-ASSESSMENT FORM

Directions: Please rate yourself from 1 to 5 on the following facilitator skills. The closer you are to a 5 within each domain, the more skilled you are at facilitation. We encourage you to complete this form prior to and after each teaching experience (e.g., a single session or an entire module). This will allow you to assess your performance as a facilitator over time.

Facilitator Behavior	1	2	3	4	5
Remains neutral					
Does not judge ideas					
Keeps the group focused on common task					
Asks clarifying questions					
Creates a climate free of criticism					
Encourages participation					
Structures participation					

Source: Adapted with permission from Welch, M. (1999). *Teaching diversity and cultural competence in health care: A trainer's guide.* San Francisco, CA: Perspectives of Differences Diversity Training and Consultation for Health Professionals (PODSDT).

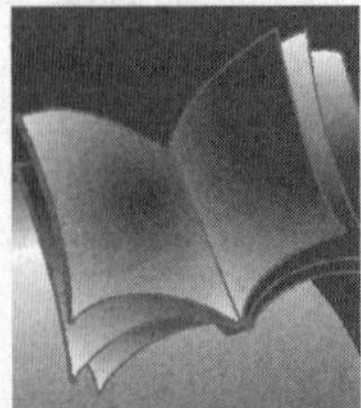

SESSION 2:

Making the Most of Teachable Moments

At the beginning of the session, the facilitator and learners should introduce themselves briefly. (If the same group has recently completed Session 1, the facilitator may decide that introductions are not needed.) Ideas for creative introductions can be found in the Facilitator's Guide.

Setting the Context: The Bright Futures Concept

(May be omitted if recently presented or when sessions are combined.)

The facilitator **(F)** introduces the learners to the Bright Futures concept of health by reading or paraphrasing the following:

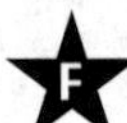 *The World Health Organization has defined health as "a state of complete physical, mental and social well-being and not merely the absence of disease or infirmity." Bright Futures embraces this broad definition of health—one that includes not only prevention of morbidity and mortality, but also the achievement of a child's full potential. In the Bright Futures concept of health, providing the capacity for healthy child development is as important as ameliorating illness or injury. Recognizing and acknowledging the strengths and resources of the child, family, and community are essential to promoting healthy growth and development.*

To build that capacity, the Pediatrics in Practice *curriculum focuses on six core concepts: Partnership, Communication, Health Promotion/Illness Prevention, Time Management, Education, and Advocacy. The curriculum also includes a companion module (Health) and videotape that present an overview of* Pediatrics in Practice *and the Bright Futures approach.*

Introducing the Session

Before introducing the session, the facilitator distributes the handout **Education: Educating Families Through Teachable Moments** to the learners. (The facilitator may choose not to distribute the handout if it was recently given to the same learners.)

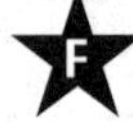 *Today's session is the second of two that comprise the* Pediatrics in Practice *Education module.*

In our last session, we discussed just how important it is for the child health professional to recognize the teachable moments that occur any time children and families are ready to learn. Using the Teachable Moments model and effective teaching strategies, we can make the most of the teachable moment.

In today's session, our objectives will be to:

▶ *Review the Teachable Moments model*

▶ *Discuss the teachable moments you've observed in your visits with children and families this week*

▶ *Use another case vignette to explore the "questioning" teaching strategy, including the use of open-ended questions and wait time*

▶ *Give you an opportunity to practice responding to a teachable moment*

When we have completed the session, you should be able to answer the following questions:

▶ *How do I partner with the child and family to begin teaching?*

▶ *How do I decide which teaching strategy (strategies) to use?*

Discussion and Exercises

The facilitator refers to the **Education: Educating Families Through Teachable Moments** handout or might display the model on a board or overhead projector and begin a very brief review of the definition of a teachable moment and the model. The review reprises the case vignette from Session 1 and offers sample questions to elicit participation.

 *A teachable moment is simply any time during the course of a health visit when the child health professional identifies an opportunity to teach the child and family. In teachable moments, the child and family are ready to learn.*

The Six-Step Teachable Moments Model

 *There are six important steps in the model. Let's go through them and review the elements of the case we discussed in Session 1.*

1. Recognize teachable moments in the health visit

 *What was the teachable moment in the last session?*

Parents Mei and Li needed to know how to use a thermometer (or Amanda needed to learn how to use a metered-dose inhaler).

2. Clarify the learning needs of the child and family

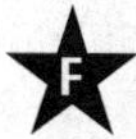 *Were the needs of the parents and pediatric provider clear?*

The needs were very clear in the vignette about the thermometer, but sometimes the needs have to be clarified.

3. Set a limited agenda and prioritize needs together

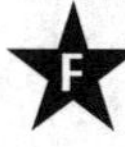 *How were the learning needs prioritized?*

Again, it was clear that the parents needed to learn how to take a temperature (or use a metered-dose inhaler). However, in those teachable moments that arise during health visits when there are many needs to be addressed and there is limited time, it is important that the family and child health professional actively participate in setting the learning priorities.

4. Select a teaching strategy

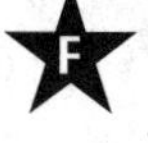 *What are the most common teaching strategies used during a health visit?*

In the last session, we discussed telling (mini-presentation), showing (demonstration), and providing resources (handouts) as appropriate teaching strategies for the teachable moment with Mei and Li. Questioning and practicing are two other appropriate strategies.

5. Seek and provide feedback

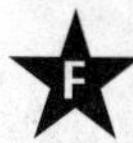 *What feedback did the pediatric provider receive?*

In the case involving the thermometer, the parents indicated both verbally and nonverbally that they understood (nodding their heads, showing recognition in their eyes).

6. Evaluate the effectiveness of the teaching

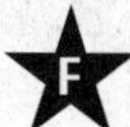 *How did the pediatric provider assess the learning that took place?*

In the last session, the pediatric provider assessed the parents' understanding by having them verbalize the instructions and demonstrate how to use the thermometer.

Optional Follow-up Exercises

[If the facilitator assigned one of the follow-up exercises suggested in Session 1, continue with the discussion that appears here under the assigned exercise. If the exercises were not assigned, disregard these discussions and go on to The Importance of Wait Time on this page.]

The facilitator continues:

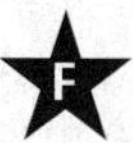 *Let's keep the Teachable Moments model in mind as we consider the exercises you were assigned at the end of the last session.*

Observation of Teachable Moments

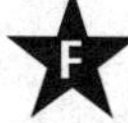 *You were asked to take notes on teachable moments during your encounters with children and families this week. You might have experienced the moment yourself, or you might have observed someone else responding to a teachable moment.*

[The facilitator might want to share some of his or her own observations, before asking the learners to share their experiences.]

The facilitator prompts the discussion with the following questions. [Not all of the questions have to be asked or answered. The objective is to get the learners to realize that once families are in the teachable moment, they are ready and often very eager to learn.]

 *Who would like to tell us about the teachable moments they experienced or observed?*

> ▶ *Who was in the encounter you observed? What was being discussed?*
>
> ▶ *What teachable moments did you observe?*
>
> ▶ *What teachable moments were missed? Why do you think so?*
>
> ▶ *Did the child health professional clarify the family's needs? How?*
>
> ▶ *Was a limited agenda set? How?*
>
> ▶ *What teaching strategies did the child health professional use?*
>
> ▶ *What would you have done differently if you were doing the teaching? Why?*
>
> ▶ *What was the most important thing you learned while completing this assignment?*

Use of Teaching Strategies

The preceding questions refer to the Observation of Teachable Moments assignment. The facilitator should ask the learners similar questions if their assignment was to practice using at least one new teaching strategy in their health visits during the week.

Review and Critique of Patient Education Materials

If the learners were assigned a review and critique of patient education materials on taking temperatures or using inhalers, the facilitator should lead a discussion of the learners' findings.

The Importance of Wait Time

The facilitator continues the session by distributing copies of the case vignette **The Polio Shot.** The learners can be invited to role-play the case, one participant can read the case aloud, or all learners can read the case silently, whichever the facilitator deems appropriate.

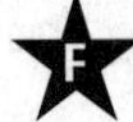 *Dr. Angelo began by asking a question about what the family knew about polio vaccines.*

He then paused or "waited" for the family's answer.

Why do you think he waited?

The facilitator invites learners' responses, which might include the following:

> ▶ The child health professional was actively listening to the family and thinking about the question. He was formulating his own question or answer in his mind.
>
> ▶ He was using the pauses to emphasize his question or response.
>
> ▶ The family was given time to reflect and consider what they were going to say, resulting in more substantive responses.

[Refer to Session 1 of the Communication module for more information on active listening.]

The facilitator continues:

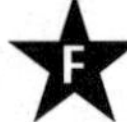 *Active listening and "wait" time are both effective strategies to use in recognizing or responding to the teachable moment.*

We are often hurried and impatient and sometimes answer or rephrase a question before a child or family has had a chance to begin to hear or process our original question. If we listen actively, we see the nonverbal cues that might tell us that the family is not ready to respond or might still be thinking about what was asked or said. Eyes averted, for example, may be a clue that the listener is still listening.

Waiting 3–5 seconds, if at all possible, before answering or rephrasing a question is always helpful, both to the listener and to the questioner. Actually counting out the time unobtrusively (one-one thousand, two-one thousand, three-one thousand, etc.) is very good practice. The pause might feel like an eternity at first, but practice is the key to becoming comfortable with the 3–5 second wait time.

Those moments of wait time might also help you to prepare a question that is clear and will ask exactly what you intend it to ask. At times child health professionals might not use any wait time and will rephrase a question immediately. Sometimes this is because they realize that their original question wasn't clear or didn't ask what they intended. Wait

Pediatrics in Practice

Practicing Wait Time

The facilitator asks the learners to break into groups of three and introduces the practice exercise:

In this exercise, we're going to learn about and practice wait time.

*During the exercise, one of you will be the **teacher**, another will be the **father**, and the third will be the **observer**. The "teacher" is seeing a 3-year-old boy who has had several ear infections. The child is in day care. The examination room smells of smoke, and the father states that he and his wife smoke outside and never around their children.*

*The teacher, aware of the teachable moment, asks a series of questions but **must wait 3–5 seconds after an answer before asking the next question**. The "father" will answer the questions, and the observer will count the wait time. After 1 minute, everyone changes roles, and after another minute roles change again so that everyone has a turn in each role.*

After all learners have had a turn in each role, the facilitator asks:

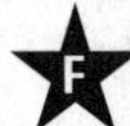

*As a **teacher**, how did it go?*

▶ *How did having to wait make you feel?*

[The facilitator should also wait 3 seconds before asking the second of the two questions.]

▶ *As the **father**, how did having the teacher wait make you feel? Did you notice?*

▶ *As an **observer**, how much time did the teacher wait after asking or answering a question?*

Although it is often difficult to wait 3–5 seconds, try to practice the wait time so that it begins to feel more comfortable to you. There may also be some times when the conversation drags because of the waiting. The increased waiting time may make the child, family, or you uncomfortable. We are all used to having a person respond relatively quickly after they have finished speaking. Use the wait time only when you think it improves your interaction with the family.

Asking Questions

The facilitator transitions to the next discussion on asking questions:

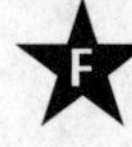

As we have seen, wait time can help the child or family to think about their response. It also gives the pediatric provider time to prepare a well-thought-out question when interviewing children and families.

Here are three steps to remember when using questions:

*1. **Prepare the question***

▶ *Ask yourself, "What is the question for?" and "Which question should I ask?"*

Different types of questions evoke different responses, as we will see in a moment.

*2. **Before you ask the question, consider how to ask it***

▶ *What is the exact wording?*

▶ *Is it open ended or closed?*

Generally, "open-ended" questions promote family-centered discussions; "closed" questions promote provider-centered discussions.

▶ *What will you do with the possible answers?*

*3. **Evaluate the question***

▶ *How effective was your question?*

▶ *Did your question do what you intended?*

Questioning Exercise

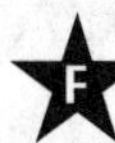

Effective questioning is both an essential communication skill and an important teaching strategy. Open-ended questions invite discussions, stimulate thinking, and are extremely helpful in identifying and responding to teachable moments.

[Refer to Session 1 of the Health Promotion module if more information on open-ended questions is needed.]

The facilitator displays the overhead for the questioning exercise.

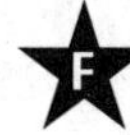

Let's look at this list of questions on the overhead. I would like you to identify whether the questions are open ended or closed and explain why.

1. Where should we begin? (**open ended**—wide range of possible answers)

2. Are Jolene's immunizations up to date? (**closed**—factual)

3. Who does Juanita see as being in her family? (**closed**—factual, small range of possible answers)

4. What makes you think that Ray is having a hard time adjusting to his new school? (**open ended**—interpretive, more qualitative)

5. What aspects of Ethan's behavior concern you the most? (**open ended**—interpretive)

6. Do you like your new neighborhood? (**closed**—yes or no answers)

7. When did Gregory's problems begin? (**closed**—factual)

8. Why do you believe that? (**open ended**—interpretive, wide range of answers)

9. What is your opinion of Morgan's social situation? (**open ended**—interpretive, more qualitative)

10. If your opinions are correct, what do you expect to happen with Jason? (**open ended**—interpretive, more qualitative)

11. What are your reactions to the problems Katrina is experiencing in her reading class? (**open ended**—interpretive)

12. What information do you have about the risks of lead poisoning? (**open ended**—range of possible answers)

13. What would happen if Tito decided not to play football this year? (**open ended**—interpretive)

14. How many teeth does Jennifer have now? (**closed**—factual)

15. What do you do when Rob refuses to do his homework? (**open ended**—range of possible answers)

The facilitator continues the discussion by asking the following questions:

 *What did you notice about the open-ended questions as a whole?*

What did you notice about the closed questions as a whole?

Open-ended questions:

▶ Tend to open up a discussion and allow changes in the direction of the discussion.

▶ Allow a broad range of acceptable responses and shared information.

Closed questions:

▶ Evoke concrete statements, facts, or yes/no answers

▶ Limit conversation and shared information

▶ Are helpful in focusing a discussion that needs direction

▶ Can help break a complicated process into manageable steps

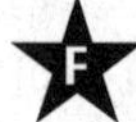 *Any discussion needs both open-ended and closed questions for everyone to understand the overall concept, to comprehend the details and facts, and to explore the potential possibilities.*

In this session, we have discussed many of the skills and strategies the child health professional can use during teachable moments. You should also be aware of some communication faults that should be avoided:

▶ Posing questions rapidly when asking factual information

▶ Waiting less than 3 seconds after posing a question

▶ Judging responses and limiting what might be said (e.g., "Good, John!")

Take-Home Message

The facilitator concludes the session:

 *Mastering any skill requires a lot of practice. It takes time before we begin to feel confident and effective.*

Every time you find yourself in an encounter with a child and/or family, try to practice at least one of the new skills we've presented in this module. In each encounter, try to recognize the teachable moment, use an appropriate teaching strategy, ask open-ended questions, and use the 3-second wait time. Before we conclude, what questions remain about what we addressed today?

Answers to the Guiding Questions

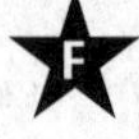 *Now that we have completed this session on Education, you should be able to answer the following questions:*

▸ How do I partner with the child and family to begin teaching?

- Speak directly to everyone and maintain eye contact
- Ask open-ended questions that invite conversation
- Pause and listen to the child and family

▸ How do I decide which teaching strategy to use?

- Clarify the learning needs of the child and family
- Set a limited agenda
- Select the strategy that best meets the needs of the child and family

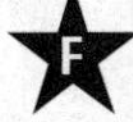 *As you leave today, please take a copy of the **Questioning and Nonquestioning Techniques** handout. This handout presents a more comprehensive examination of communication skills and can serve as a helpful reference for you as you practice using the skills we've covered in this module.*

Evaluation

The facilitator now distributes the **Session Evaluation Form**, the **Preceptor Structured Observation Form**, and the **Patient and Family Survey Form**. The facilitator also completes the **Facilitator Self-Assessment Form**.

Modifications to Session 2 (if presented without Session 1)

If Session 2 is presented without Session 1, Session 2 is adjusted to incorporate more information about the Teachable Moments model. The remainder of the session focuses on questioning as a communication skill and a teaching strategy and includes a practice exercise on wait time.

Introduction

The facilitator might consider using or paraphrasing the following:

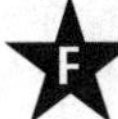 *Today, I am going to show you a model that you can use any time in health encounters with children and families. It is called "Teachable Moments." When I say teachable moments, what do you think that is?*

The facilitator invites responses from the learners. The facilitator then distributes the **Education: Educating Families Through Teachable Moments** handout and may display the model on an overhead projector. The facilitator continues with the session.

Definition

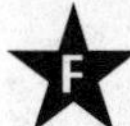 *A teachable moment is simply any time during the course of a health visit when the child health professional identifies an opportunity to teach the child and family. Teachable moments are those when the child and family are ready to learn.*

The Six-Step Teachable Moments Model

1. **Recognize** "teachable moments."
2. **Assess.** Clarify the needs of the child and/or family.
3. **Plan.** Set a limited agenda and prioritize needs together.
4. **Implement.** Select a teaching strategy to meet the needs (telling, showing, providing resources, practicing, questioning, and giving feedback).
5. **Feedback.** Seek and provide feedback.
6. **Evaluation.** Assess the effectiveness of the teaching.

After that brief review of the model, the facilitator continues:

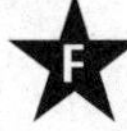 *Let me give you a nonmedical example:*

Raminda is at the checkout stand at the grocery store, and the young clerk points to an avocado and says, "Is this an artichoke or an avocado?" Raminda replies, "It's an avocado. Avocados are pear shaped with very wrinkly dark green skin. An artichoke is about the size of an orange or grapefruit and looks like a big flower before its petals are open."

In this scenario, Raminda:

▸ *Recognized the teachable moment. The clerk had a need to know the difference between the avocado and the artichoke.*

▸ *Didn't clarify the clerk's learning needs more, but assumed he didn't recognize the physical differences between the two vegetables.*

▸ *Limited the agenda to answering his question directly.*

▶ Used the teaching strategy of "telling" him what the physical differences were.

▶ Realized he had understood by his nodding to her, smiling, and ringing up the right price.

▶ Did all of this in about 10 seconds.

The teachable moment has certain characteristics. A teachable moment:

▶ Provides "information bites" or small amounts of information (the physical differences in the vegetables).

▶ Is directed to an individual or a small group (the clerk).

▶ Is brief (lasts just a few seconds).

▶ Requires no preparation time (Raminda already knew the answer).

The facilitator can then proceed with Session 2 as presented earlier.

Education: Session 2

EDUCATION: EDUCATING FAMILIES THROUGH TEACHABLE MOMENTS

A teachable moment is simply any time during the course of a health visit when the child health professional identifies an opportunity to teach the child and family. Teachable moments are the moments when the child and family are ready to learn.

1. Recognize "teachable moments" in health visit

2. Clarify learning needs of child and family

3. Set a limited agenda and prioritize needs together

4. Select teaching strategy

5. Seek and provide feedback

6. Evaluate effectiveness of teaching

Four characteristics of the teachable moment
- Provides "information bites" (small amounts of information)
- Is directed to the child's or family's specific need
- Is brief (e.g., a few seconds)
- Requires no preparation time

Teaching strategies	**Advantages**
■ Telling (explain, provide information, give directions)	Works well when giving initial explanations or clarifying concepts
■ Showing (demonstrate, model, draw)	Illustrates concepts for visual learners
■ Providing resources (handouts, videos, Web sites)	Serves as reference after family leaves the office/clinic
■ Questioning (ask open-ended questions, allow time for response)	Promotes problem-solving, critical thinking; elicits better information; stimulates recall
■ Practicing (apply new information)	Reinforces new concepts
■ Giving constructive feedback (seek family's perspective, correct misunderstandings, restate, clarify)	Affirms family's knowledge; corrects misunderstandings

Source: Reproduced with permission from Green. M., Palfrey, J.S., Clark, E.M., & Anastasi, J.M. (Eds.) (2002). *Bright futures: Guidelines for health supervision of infants, children, and adolescents* (2nd ed., rev.)—*Pocket guide.* Arlington, VA: National Center for Education in Maternal and Child Health.

Education: Session 2

CASE VIGNETTE: THE POLIO SHOT

Dr. Angelo, a third-year resident in continuity clinic, is concluding a well-baby visit with 2-month-old Beth and her parents. He has just finished discussing the immunizations Beth will receive today.

> **Dr. Angelo:** What questions do you have about the shots Beth will get today?
>
> **Paul** (father, appearing slightly confused): Why is she getting a polio shot?
>
> **Sue** (mother, also appearing slightly confused): Yes. Our older daughter just had a drink.

Dr. Angelo pauses, leans slightly forward in his chair.

> **Dr. Angelo:** What do you know about the polio vaccines?
>
> **Paul:** Well, when I was growing up, we all got a drink. I know that there's not much polio around any more.

Dr. Angelo again pauses before continuing.

> **Dr. Angelo:** That's right. There is less polio now because of the vaccines' success. There are two kinds of polio vaccines: a drink and a shot. All vaccines carry some risk, and children who receive the drink have a slight risk of developing polio. The polio shot eliminates that risk. That's why it's the only kind of vaccine we use in this country now to prevent polio.
>
> **Sue** (still concerned): Can't Beth still have the drink? She's already getting so many shots today.

Dr. Angelo again pauses.

> **Dr. Angelo:** Is Beth around anyone who has problems fighting infections, uses steroid medicines, or has cancer or AIDS?
>
> **Sue:** Oh, yes. My mother is using steroids and she helps us out a lot with babysitting.
>
> **Dr. Angelo:** That's another reason to use the polio shot. The drink vaccine could increase the risk to your mother and possibly make her sick.
>
> **Paul:** So if the shot has fewer risks and won't make Grandma sick, then it's an easy choice. Beth has to have the shot.

Education: Session 2

QUESTIONING AND NONQUESTIONING TECHNIQUES

Asking Questions, Not Giving Answers

The questions you ask as a health professional help to direct the discussion among you, your patients, and their families. They also help move the focus away from you. Your questions not only facilitate the discussion or health interview, but they also convey your interest in the child and family.

Open a discussion with a "starter" question such as: "How are you?" or "Where would you like to begin?" These questions are valuable in eliciting the needs and concerns of the child or family.

Enrich the discussion with questions that allow a broad range of appropriate responses. Changing the types of questions you ask often helps to advance to a family-centered discussion.

Identify the most appropriate types of questions to facilitate a family-centered discussion. There are **seven general types of questions** listed below that a health professional might ask the family. They can help move the discussion from the general to the specific or vice versa.

1. **Diagnosis:** "What do you think is going on?" "What makes you think that way?"

2. **Action:** "Where should we begin?" "What aspects of your child's problem(s) are of greatest interest to you?"

3. **Information Gathering:** "Who is in Armando's family?" "When did you first become aware of the problem?"

4. **Challenge:** "Why do you believe that?" "What supports your thinking?"

5. **Extension:** "How is his behavior related to his grades?" "How is the symptom related to the diagnosis?"

6. **Prediction:** "What problems do you see with trying to follow this plan?" "How do you anticipate your child reacting to this course of treatment?"

7. **Generalization:** "Based upon your child's diagnosis, do you recognize these symptoms/behaviors in your other children at home?" "How do you think Ethan is talking compared to other children his age?"

(continued on next page)

Education: Session 2

QUESTIONING AND NONQUESTIONING TECHNIQUES (continued)

The Use of Questions

When asking questions, it is important to keep the following points in mind:

Prepare the question
- Ask yourself *"What is the question for?"* and *"Which question should I ask?"*
- Consider the different types of questions you might use.

Consider how to ask the question
- Before you ask the question, decide if it should be an open-ended or closed question. Consider what you will do with the answer.

  Generally, open-ended questions promote family-centered discussion; closed questions promote provider-centered discussion.

  Open-ended: What you do with your friends to have fun?

  Closed: Do you have any friends?

Evaluate the question
- How effective were your questions?
- Did your questions do what you intended?

Nonquestioning Techniques

There are many types of questions that can be asked, but questions combined with statements and silence (nonquestioning techniques) all contribute to and promote learning.

   Other useful techniques include:

Silence
- An important aspect of **listening.**

Five important areas of listening
- Listen for:
  - **Content, logic, substantive facts, intellectual information.** This is what is most obvious.
  - **Continuity.** Listen over time to observe change. Remember what was said, and in what context, so that you can refer back later to what was said.
  - **Mechanics.** Which words are spoken loudly, and which are mumbled?

(continued on next page)

Education: Session 2

QUESTIONING AND NONQUESTIONING TECHNIQUES (continued)

Five important areas of listening (*continued*)	• A person's **capacity** to listen. Is the parent distracted?
	
	• **Emotion**, especially:
	   a. *certitude:* absolutes or conditionals used
	   b. *depth of feeling:* voice tone, spoken words, and latent feelings

Statements	• **Declarative.** "I think the problem is X." • **Reflective.** Repeating what has been said (stating again in the same form) and restating (stating again in a different or summary form).
Referral	• **"Linking"** or stating the relationship between what the child/family has just said and what the previous speaker said.
Polling	• **Posing the topic** to other members of the group. "Let's take a minute to hear what someone else is thinking" (most useful in teaching).

Improving Interviews with Children and Families

In interviews with children and families, discussion improves when:

- The pediatric provider speaks calmly and gives the child or family time to consider and answer questions.

- The pediatric provider waits for 3–5 seconds after asking a question.

- The pediatric provider responds in a nonjudgmental manner.

- The pediatric provider asks questions that encourage the child or family to demonstrate that they understand what has been said.

Education: Session 2

SESSION EVALUATION FORM

Session 2: Making the Most of Teachable Moments

Date: _______________________________

Facilitator(s): _______________________________

Site: _______________________________

1. Overall, I found the "Making the Most of Teachable Moments" session to be:

Not Useful			Very Useful	
1	2	3	4	5

2. The objectives of the session were:

Not Clear				Clear
1	2	3	4	5

3. The organization of the session was:

Poor				Excellent
1	2	3	4	5

4. The communication skills of the facilitator(s) were:

Poor				Excellent
1	2	3	4	5

5. The facilitator(s) stimulated interest in the subject matter:

Not at All			Very Much	
1	2	3	4	5

6. The facilitator(s) encouraged group participation:

Not at All			Very Much	
1	2	3	4	5

7. Handouts or visual aids (if used) were:

Not Helpful		Very Helpful		
1	2	3	4	5

8. Any additional comments?

____
____
____

9. The most useful features of the session were:

____
____
____

10. Suggestions for improvement

____
____
____

11. Suggestions for topics related to this session

____
____
____

Education: Session 2

PRECEPTOR STRUCTURED OBSERVATION FORM

Effective Behaviors Using the Teachable Moments Model			
Behavior	Observed	Not Observed	Not Applicable
Recognizes "teachable moments" in the health visit			
Clarifies the learning needs of the child and family			
Sets a limited agenda and prioritizes learning needs with the child and family			
Selects appropriate teaching strategy			
Uses teaching materials appropriately (e.g., handouts)			
Seeks feedback from and provides feedback to the child and family			
Evaluates effectiveness of teaching			
Uses teaching time appropriately during the health visit			

Comments

____

____

____

____

____

____

____

____

____

Education: Session 2

PATIENT AND FAMILY SURVEY FORM

To our Patients and Families:

The child health professionals in our clinic are very interested in your opinions about the care that we provide for you and your child. As part of our effort to continue to improve the care we offer, we ask that you please complete this survey about today's visit. Your responses will be confidential and will not be shared directly with your child health professional.

Thank you for your time in completing this survey.

The Staff of the Clinic

PATIENT AND FAMILY SURVEY	I am a: ☐ Patient ☐ Family Member				
My Child Health Professional:	Disagree <—> Uncertain <—> Agree				
Recognized that I wanted to learn more about an issue	1	2	3	4	5
Helped me to make clear what I wanted to learn	1	2	3	4	5
Helped me to talk about the most important issues first	1	2	3	4	5
Gave me the information clearly so I could understand it	1	2	3	4	5
Asked me what I did or did not understand	1	2	3	4	5
Gave me enough time to talk about my concerns	1	2	3	4	5

Comments

____

____

____

____

____

____

____

____

____

Education: Session 2

QUESTIONING EXERCISE

1. Where should we begin?

2. Are Jolene's immunizations up to date?

3. Who does Juanita see as being in her family?

4. What makes you think that Ray is having a hard time adjusting to his new school?

5. What aspects of Ethan's behavior concern you the most?

6. Do you like your new neighborhood?

7. When did Gregory's problems begin?

8. Why do you believe that?

9. What is your opinion of Morgan's social situation?

10. If your opinions are correct, what do you expect to happen with Jason?

11. What are your reactions to the problems Katrina is experiencing in her reading class?

12. What information do you have about the risks of lead poisoning?

13. What would happen if Tito decided not to play football this year?

14. How many teeth does Jennifer have now?

15. What do you do when Rob refuses to do his homework?

Education: Session 2

FACILITATOR SELF-ASSESSMENT FORM

Directions: Please rate yourself from 1 to 5 on the following facilitator skills. The closer you are to a 5 within each domain, the more skilled you are at facilitation. We encourage you to complete this form prior to and after each teaching experience (e.g., a single session or an entire module). This will allow you to assess your performance as a facilitator over time.

Facilitator Behavior	1	2	3	4	5
Remains neutral					
Does not judge ideas					
Keeps the group focused on common task					
Asks clarifying questions					
Creates a climate free of criticism					
Encourages participation					
Structures participation					

Source: Adapted with permission from Welch, M. (1999). *Teaching diversity and cultural competence in health care: A trainer's guide.* San Francisco, CA: Perspectives of Differences Diversity Training and Consultation for Health Professionals (PODSDT).

References

Benjamin, J.T., Cimino, S.A., & Hafler, J.P., Bright Futures Health Promotion Work Group, & Bernstein, H.H. (2002). The office visit: A time to promote health—but how? *Contemporary Pediatrics, 19*(2), 90–107.

Christensen, C.R., Garvin, D.A., & Sweet, A. (1991). *Education for judgment: The artistry of discussion leadership.* Boston, MA: Harvard Business School Press.

Green, M., & Palfrey, J.S., (Eds.) (2002). *Bright futures: Guidelines for health supervision of infants, children, and adolescents* (2nd ed., rev.). Arlington, VA: National Center for Education in Maternal and Child Health.

Green, M., Palfrey, J.S., Clark, E.M., & Anastasi, J.M., (Eds.) (2002). *Bright futures: Guidelines for health supervision of infants, children, and adolescents* (2nd ed., rev.)—*Pocket guide.* Arlington, VA: National Center for Education in Maternal and Child Health.

Lesky, L.G., Borkan, S.C. (1990). Strategies to improve teaching in the ambulatory medicine setting. *Archives of Internal Medicine, 150,* 2133–2137.

Napell, S.M.. (1976). Six common non-facilitating teaching behaviors. *Contemporary Education, 47*(2), 79–82.

Neher, G., & Meyer, S. (1992). A five-step microskills model of clinical teaching. *Journal of the American Board of Family Practice, 5,* 419–424.

Skeff, K. (1998). Enhancing teaching effectiveness and vitality in the ambulatory setting. *Journal of General Internal Medicine, 123,* S26–S33.

Stritter, F.T., Baker, R.M., & Shadady, E.J. (1986). Clinical instruction. In McGaghie, W.C., & Frey, J.J., (Eds.) *Handbook for the academic physician.* New York: Springer-Verlag.

Resources

Adult Learning Principles and Clinical Teaching

Spencer, P.E., & Alden, E. (1996). Educational foundations for community-based programs. In DeWitt, T.G., Roberts, K.B., (Eds.) *Pediatric dducation in community settings: A manual,* p. 14. Arlington, VA: National Center for Education in Maternal and Child Health.

Weinholtz, D., & Edwards, J. (1991). *Teaching during rounds: A handbook for attending physicians and learners.* Baltimore, MD: Johns Hopkins Press.

Whitman N, Schwenk T. 1997. *The Physician As Teacher* (2nd ed.), pp. 33–37. Salt Lake City, UT: Whitman Associates.

Other Clinical Teaching Models (similar to the "Teachable Moments" model)

McGee, S.R., & Irby, D.M. (1997). Teaching in the outpatient clinic: Practical tips. *Journal of General Internal Medicine, 12,* S34–S40.

Educational, Psychological, and Theory

Arceneau, R., & Rodenburg, D. (1998). The developmental perspective. In Pratt, D.D., & Malabar, F.L., (Eds.) *Five perspectives on teaching in adult and higher education.* Melbourne, FL: Kreiger Publications.

Brown, J.S., Collins, A., & Duguid, P. (1989). Situated cognition and the culture of learning. *Educational Researcher, 18*(1), 32–42.

Dillon, J.T. (1990). *The practice of questioning.* London: Routledge.

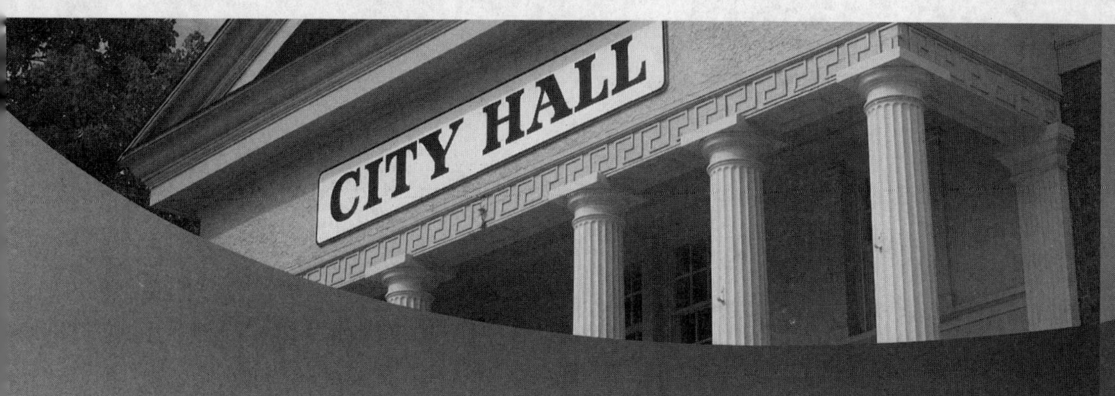

Chapter 8

Advocacy

Advocating for Children, Families, and Communities

Judith S. Shaw

Emily J. Roth

Richard Pan

Danielle Laraque

CONTENTS

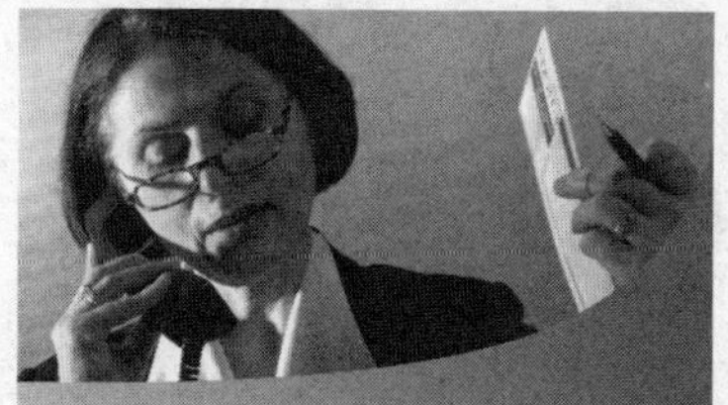

ADVOCACY
Advocating for Children, Families, and Communities

OVERVIEW

Background

Child health professionals have the unique opportunity to practice advocacy each day they interact with children and families. They can be involved in child advocacy either at an individual level (accessing information or services for a child or family) or at a local or national level (sharing information with the community, disseminating information through the media, and speaking out in support of a legislative issue). Although the voices of child health professionals can have a profound impact on a child or family's ability to obtain services, or on local and national policies, most child health professionals lack formal training in advocacy.

Goal

The overall goal of this module is to expand the role of child health professionals to include advocacy by helping them develop the knowledge, skills, and attitudes they need to become effective advocates for children and families within their communities.

This module will enable learners to:

▶ Apply a four-step approach to advocating on behalf of an individual or a group at a local or national level

▶ Identify available resources to support child advocacy

Instructional Design

This module consists of two 30-minute sessions.

▶ Session 1 delineates advocacy and presents a four-step approach to advocacy on an individual level.

▶ Session 2 applies the four-step approach to advocacy on behalf of a group or community.

▶ Each of the two sessions can be used as a separate, stand-alone offering, or the sessions can be combined. See the Facilitator's Guide for information on combining sessions.

▶ If Session 1 is not presented, the explanation of the effective use of interview questions (see Session 1) should be expanded in Session 2.

▶ Though written case vignettes are provided for this module, it is also possible to use a real situation presented by one of the learners.

▶ Learners may also choose an advocacy issue they would like to explore together and use this model to plan their project.

Teaching Strategies

The teaching strategies used in this module include case discussion and brainstorming. These strategies have been selected to help learners develop the skills required to advocate effectively on behalf of individuals and groups. Please refer to the Facilitator's Guide for more information related to each strategy.

Evaluation

Learners will complete a **Session Evaluation Form** and a **Learner Self-Assessment Form** following each session. Facilitators are encouraged to complete a **Facilitator Self-Assessment Form** prior to and following each teaching experience (e.g., a single session or an entire module) in order to assess their performance over time.

Guiding Questions

Learners who have completed the entire Advocacy module should be able to answer the following questions:

▶ What are the essential elements of advocacy?

▶ How do open-ended questions facilitate identification of child, parent, or family concerns?

▶ How do I, as a pediatric provider, determine where and how to focus my advocacy efforts?

INTRODUCTION TO TEACHING SESSIONS

Session 1: Advocating for the Needs of an Individual

Objectives

The objectives for this session are for the facilitator to:

▶ Define advocacy as it applies to the child health professional

▶ Describe the four-step approach to advocacy

▶ Allow the learners to practice the four-step approach by planning how to advocate for a child and/or family

Materials

The materials and teaching aids needed for this session are:

Handouts

▶ Advocacy: Advocating for Children, Families, and Communities

▶ Defining Advocacy and Other Related Terms

▶ Stepwise: The Four-Step Approach to Advocacy

▶ Case Vignette: Taylor's Learning Problems

▶ Session Evaluation Form

▶ Learner Self-Assessmenr Form

Facilitator Form

▶ Facilitator Self-Assessment Form

Teaching Aids

▶ Display board, flip chart, or chalkboard

▶ Markers or chalk

Time

The time allocated for this session is 30 minutes.

Session 2: Advocating for the Needs of a Group

Objectives

The objectives for this session are for the facilitator to:

▶ Review and reinforce the four-step approach to advocacy

▶ Allow the learners to practice the four-step approach by planning how to advocate for the needs of a group on a local or national level

Materials

The materials and teaching aids needed for this session are:

Handouts

▶ Advocacy: Advocating for Children, Families, and Communities

▶ Stepwise: The Four-Step Approach to Advocacy

▶ Case Vignette: John's Emergency Department Visit

▶ Session Evaluation Form

▶ Learner Self-Assessment Form

Facilitator Form

▶ Facilitator Self-Assessment Form

Teaching Aids

▶ Display board, flip chart, or chalkboard

▶ Markers or chalk

Time

The time allocated for this session is 30 minutes.

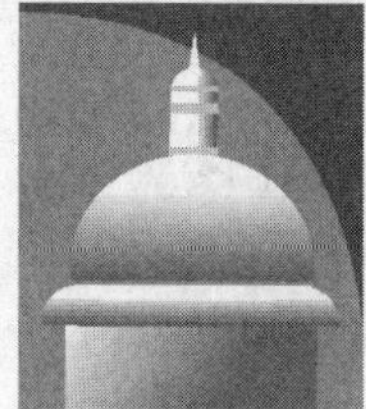

SESSION 1:
Advocating for the Needs of an Individual

At the beginning of the session, the facilitator and learners should introduce themselves briefly. Ideas for creative introductions can be found in the Facilitator's Guide.

Setting the Context: The Bright Futures Concept

The facilitator **(F)** introduces the learners to the Bright Futures concept of health by reading or paraphrasing the following:

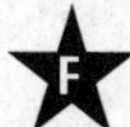 *The World Health Organization has defined health as "a state of complete physical, mental and social well-being and not merely the absence of disease or infirmity." Bright Futures embraces this broad definition of health—one that includes not only prevention of morbidity and mortality, but also the achievement of a child's full potential. In the Bright Futures concept of health, providing the capacity for healthy child development is as important as ameliorating illness or injury. Recognizing and acknowledging the strengths and resources of the child, family, and community are essential to promoting healthy growth and development.*

To build that capacity, the Pediatrics in Practice *curriculum focuses on six core concepts: Partnership, Communication, Health Promotion/Illness Prevention, Time Management, Education, and Advocacy. The curriculum also includes a companion module (Health) and videotape that present an overview of* Pediatrics in Practice *and the Bright Futures approach.*

Introducing the Session

Before introducing the session, the facilitator distributes the handout **Advocacy: Advocating for Children, Families, and Communities** to the learners.

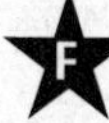 *Today's session is the first of two that comprise the* Pediatrics in Practice *Advocacy module. Your* **Advocacy: Advocating for Children, Families, and Communities** *handout outlines the steps involved in advocating for children, families, and communities. We will cover these steps in more detail as we go through today's session.*

Child health professionals have the unique opportunity to practice advocacy each day they interact with children and families. They can be involved in child advocacy either at an individual level (accessing information or services for a child or family) or at a local or national level (sharing information with the community, disseminating information through the media, and speaking out in support of a legislative issue). Although the voices of child health professionals can have a profound impact on a child or family's ability to obtain services, or on local and national policies, most pediatric providers lack formal training in advocacy.

In today's session, our objectives will be to:

▶ *Define advocacy as it pertains to you, the child health professional*

▶ *Introduce the four-step approach to advocacy*

▶ *Practice using the four-step approach to advocate for a child or family*

The session will have two parts:

▶ *Deciding what to advocate for*

▶ *Applying the four-step approach*

When we have completed the session, you should be able to answer the following questions:

▶ *What are the essential elements of advocacy?*

▶ *How do open-ended questions facilitate identification of child, parent, or family concerns?*

Discussion and Exercises

Defining Advocacy

The facilitator distributes the **Defining Advocacy and Other Related Terms** handout and asks:

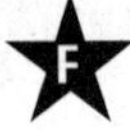 *How would you define "advocacy"? Suggest some words that come to mind when you hear the phrase "to advocate" or the word "advocacy."*

At the display board or flip chart, the facilitator begins a list from the learners' suggestions. If suggestions are slow in coming, one or two of the following can be used to prompt further ideas from the learners.

Plead	Protect	A cause
Argue	Defend	An idea
Support	Take a stand	A policy
Attitude	Belief	Uphold
Opinion	Assist	Reason
Debate	Help	Sustain

After noting the suggestions, the facilitator continues:

 *The American Heritage Dictionary defines advocacy as the act of pleading or arguing in favor of something, such as a cause, an idea, or a policy; active support.*

Deciding What to Advocate For

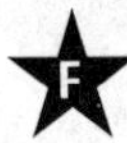 *There are many ways to define the term "advocacy," but in order to be an advocate for a child and family at any level, the child health professional must know for what he or she is advocating. In the case of an individual patient and family, the process begins by interviewing the child and family to elicit their true needs and concerns.*

Gathering Information

The facilitator continues:

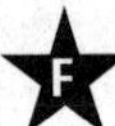 *Some of you may already be familiar with the use of interview questions to elicit a child and family's needs or concerns. For you, the following will be a brief refresher. For others, this will emphasize a few important points to remember when asking interview questions.*

The facilitator writes the following on the display board:

▶ All questions should be nonjudgmental.

▶ Open-ended questions support a dialogue between the child and/or family and the pediatric provider, and often elicit the family's needs and concerns.

▶ Yes/no answers can provide important information, particularly in follow-up to open-ended questions.

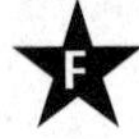 *Here are some questions that might prove useful when interviewing the child and family:*

The facilitator reads or writes the following:

1. What are some of the main concerns in your life right now? Do they include transportation? Housing? Personal safety? What assistance would be helpful with these issues?

2. Tell me about your neighborhood. How safe is it?

3. How much time do you have for yourself? Who helps you with your child (children)?

4. What are some of the things you worry about?

5. When you ride your bicycle, rollerblade, or skateboard, what protective equipment do you use? Do you wear a helmet?

6. Does anyone in your home have a gun? How do you store it? Is it unloaded and locked up? Where is the ammunition stored? Have you considered removing the gun from your home?

7. Does anyone smoke in your house?

8. What concerns do you have about health insurance for your children?

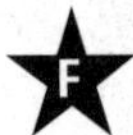 *Open-ended questions help to elicit the child and/or family's true needs and concerns. This is an important step in creating advocacy priorities. The next part of this session will provide a stepwise approach that can be used to navigate the advocacy process.*

Stepwise: The Four-Step Approach to Advocacy

This part of the session introduces the four-step approach to advocacy. The facilitator can either present these four steps to the group, followed by a discussion of the case, or can introduce each step and apply the case as the discussion moves along.

The facilitator distributes the handouts **Stepwise: The Four-Step Approach to Advocacy** and **Case Vignette: Taylor's Learning Problems.** The facilitator begins as follows:

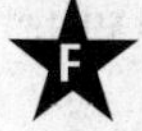

I have distributed two handouts. One outlines the four-step approach to answering the question "How do I advocate for a child, family, and/or community?"

The other handout is a case vignette. We will use the four-step approach to organize our response to the problem raised in the vignette. Would one of you please read the vignette aloud to the group?

Using the display board or flip chart, the facilitator introduces the first step in the Stepwise approach and its supporting activities:

STEP 1: Identify Family Needs or Concerns

a. Use open-ended questions to identify specific family needs or concerns

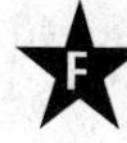

Using open-ended question/comments, gather specific information about the learning difficulties that Taylor's mother feels her daughter is having. What are some questions you might ask?

Examples:

▶ Please describe for me specifically what you have observed when Taylor reads and writes.

▶ Please describe Taylor's teacher's assessment of her progress in school. Have you discussed your concerns with the teacher?

▶ What was stated in her report card or end-of-year report from last year?

▶ What support have you received from the school's evaluation team?

▶ Please describe any signs of stress that Taylor has shown lately. Has she been experiencing any other difficulties at school or at home?

▶ Please describe the difficulties that Taylor may have paying attention at school. Have you noticed this at home?

b. Choose a specific area of focus

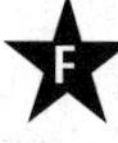

In this case, what is the primary problem that Taylor needs help with? (Reading and writing.) She and her family might also benefit from someone to advocate on their behalf with school personnel, such as the teacher or special education staff.

When advocating on an individual, community, or national level, identifying the specific problems is important to making effective change.

c. Clarify the family's beliefs and expectations about the issue

What does the family believe is the cause of the problem? What expectations do they have for Taylor? What expectations do they have of you in helping them address this problem?

Understanding the child and parent's beliefs and expectations helps to clarify how they view the problem.

You might ask the following:

▶ What are you concerned about the most?

▶ Why do you think Taylor is having more trouble with reading and writing?

▶ How do the books that Taylor is reading compare with what other children in her class are reading?

▶ What would you like to see Taylor reading or writing at this time?

▶ What else can I do to assist you at this time?

▶ Taylor, what do you enjoy about school?

▶ How do you feel about your school work this year?

d. Determine what has been done to date and what has (or has not) worked

From your questions and information gathering let us say you have determined:

▶ *Taylor's reading and writing have not progressed from last year. In fact, her mother feels she is falling farther and farther behind. Her mother notes that she reads very slowly and is unable to recall what she has read. She has difficulty reading all but the simplest words.*

▶ *Taylor is not getting any services through the school. The teacher suggested that Taylor's issues were behavioral and not a learning disability.*

e. Do some initial "fact finding" and obtain data

 *Your assessment of the situation should include gathering additional information. You might obtain the following "data" or "facts."*

- ▶ Attention rating forms completed by Taylor's teachers and parents
- ▶ Taylor's report card from last year
- ▶ Her behavior at school and at home

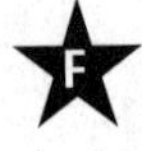 *According to her mother, Taylor has not demonstrated any behavioral problems or signs of inattention at school or at home, but her attention during reading declines.*

- ▶ Other factors that might affect Taylor's reading or writing

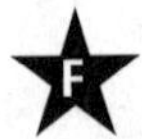 *You discover that her vision and hearing screening are normal.*

f. Talk with others, determine progress to date on the issue

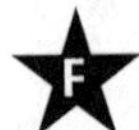 *Speaking with others, such as Taylor's teacher, may provide additional information.*

STEP 2: Assess the Situation

a. Determine existing community resources

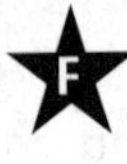 *Based on the specific need or concern you have identified and explored, the next step is to develop a list of possible resources to address the need.*

Examples:

- ▶ What remedial services are available from the school itself?
- ▶ What are the possibilities for referrals to other professionals?
- ▶ What might Taylor's health plan provide?
- ▶ What other child-focused services might be available?
- ▶ What services are available in your own clinic?

b. Learn the laws

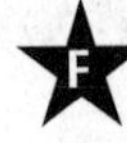 *Is there a law that covers what you are advocating for? If so, what resources does the legislation provide? You might want to consult a local social worker or the legal aid society to learn about the laws that pertain to the issue you are advocating for.*

For example:

The Individuals with Disabilities Education Act requires public school systems to provide special education services to children with disabilities who are 3 years and older. Familiarity with laws regarding special education and other services can be very useful.

c. Review the data and resources

 *Document the problem to be sure it supports the issue.*

In this case:

- ▶ Verify that Taylor's report card shows evidence of a remedial need.
- ▶ Talk with Taylor's teacher to determine if he/she might acknowledge that the problem is not a behavioral one.
- ▶ Ask for the teacher's support in seeking remedial services for Taylor.

d. Assess the political or service climate

 *Is this issue of interest to anyone else (a school administrator, the teacher, a local policymaker)? Who or what might oppose you in your advocacy efforts and why?*

For example:

Are the special education service providers underfunded and/or overwhelmed?

STEP 3: Develop a Strategy

a. Limit efforts to a specific issue

 *While there may be other patient or family issues that warrant attention, it is best to stay focused on one area at a time.*

In this case, helping Taylor with reading and writing is the chosen issue.

b. Use existing resources

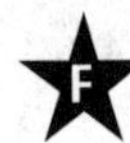 *At this point, you should begin to develop your action plan using existing resources. In this example, what strategies might be used?*

Efforts might include:

Requesting services from the school

- ▶ Write a letter to the school district documenting Taylor's issues and request an evaluation for special education services.
- ▶ Call the school to discuss Taylor's needs with her teacher, and ask him/her to join in the request for an evaluation.

- ▶ Attend Taylor's special education evaluation meeting at the school.
- ▶ Plan a follow-up visit in your office after the evaluation is complete. Discuss the findings and the resources offered.

Making referrals to other community resources

- ▶ Explore the option of obtaining an evaluation or support at a community-based center (e.g., center for language and learning or communications disorder center).
- ▶ Refer Taylor's family to a social worker or case manager who can help the family access services in the community.
- ▶ Discuss the possibility of Taylor's family obtaining support (or an advocate) from a community or national support group (e.g., Federation for Children with Special Health Care Needs).

Using the health care system

- ▶ Help the family obtain therapy and other services through their health coverage.

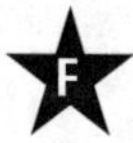 *Prioritize your action plan based on resources that are most easily attainable. In our example, what would be the best place to begin?*

1. Seek services from the school.
2. Make referral to other professionals (this could take time based on case load and available resources).
3. Use the health care system (the family may have no or limited coverage).

c. Start with small steps and build upon success

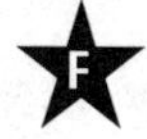 *In what order would you request services from the school?*

1. Contact the teacher again.
2. Write a letter to the school district.
3. Attend the special education evaluation.

STEP 4: Follow Through

a. Be passionate about the issue

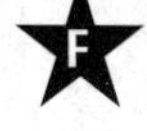 *Commit yourself to the problem or need, but be willing to negotiate.*

b. Review the outcome

 *Keep abreast of and reexamine the different steps in your action plan as you take them.*

c. Evaluate your efforts

 *Reflect on your effort to date. Ask yourself the following questions:*

- ▶ Have I addressed the family's primary concern?
- ▶ What worked, what didn't work, and why?
- ▶ What else needs to be done?

d. Determine next steps in partnership with the family

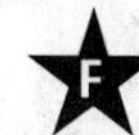 *Partner with the family to determine what the next steps might be.*

Example:

- ▶ Determine how you and the family will track Taylor's progress following your intervention.
- ▶ Using open-ended questions, ask Taylor and her family what they believe should be the next steps in providing support for Taylor's reading and writing.

e. Recognize that child health professionals and families can learn from one another about effective advocacy

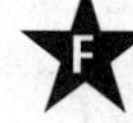 *Accessing services for children and families, especially those outside the medical system, can be confusing for both the family and the pediatric provider. You and the family can learn from one another about how to effectively advocate for children and their needs.*

Take-Home Message

The facilitator ends the session with the following:

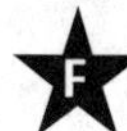 *This session has provided a basic introduction to advocacy by defining it, teaching a four-step approach to advocacy, and applying these steps to a case. I hope this session has illustrated how a relatively small effort on your part can have a large impact on a child or family's life. Before we conclude, what questions remain about what we addressed today?*

Answers to the Guiding Questions

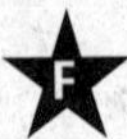 *Now that we have completed this session on Advocacy, you should be able to answer the following questions:*

- ▶ What are the essential elements of advocacy?
  - Identifying child or family needs or concerns, assessing the situation, developing a strategy, and following through with it.
- ▶ How do open-ended questions facilitate identification of child/family concerns?
  - Open-ended questions support a dialogue between the child and/or family and the pediatric provider and often elicit the needs or concerns of the family.

Planning for the Next Session (if Session 2 is planned)

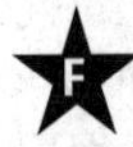 *At the next session, we will apply the four-step approach to either another vignette or an actual case to demonstrate how to effectively advocate for the needs of a group at the local/national level.*

To prepare for the next session, the facilitator asks the learners to consider the following question:

- ▶ How do I, as a pediatric provider, determine where and how to focus my advocacy efforts?

Evaluation

The facilitator now distributes the **Session Evaluation Form** and the **Learner Self-Assessment Form.** The facilitator also completes the **Facilitator Self-Assessment Form.**

Advocacy: Session 1

ADVOCACY: ADVOCATING FOR CHILDREN, FAMILIES, AND COMMUNITIES

Health professionals can be involved in advocacy either at an individual level (for example, obtaining services for a child or family) or at a local or national level (speaking with the media, community groups, or legislators).

1. Identify Family Needs or Concerns.
- Use open-ended questions to identify specific needs or concerns of the family
  Example: "What are some of the main concerns in your life right now?"
- Choose a specific area of focus
  Example: Obtaining special education services for a child.
- Clarify family's beliefs and expectations about the issue
- Determine what has been done to date, and what has (or hasn't) worked
  Example: Parents may have tried unsuccessfully to obtain services for their child.
- Do some initial "fact finding" and obtain data
  Example: Contact board of education or local department of public health.
- Talk with others, determine progress
  Example: Is there a local school coalition that addresses the issue?

2. Assess the Situation.
- Determine existing community resources
- Learn the laws
  Example: Are there any existing laws that address the issue?
- Review the data and resources to be sure they support the issue
- Assess political climate to determine support or opposition
  Example: Is this issue of interest to anyone else (school/early intervention teacher, local policymakers)? Who (or what) might oppose the advocacy efforts? Why?

3. Develop a Strategy.
- Limit efforts to a specific issue
  Example: Obtaining special education services for a child rather than changing the laws.
- Use existing resources
- Start with small steps, then build upon successes
  Examples: Write a letter to the school district. Attend the special education evaluation.

4. Follow Through.
- Be passionate about the issue, but willing to negotiate
- Review the outcome
- Evaluate your efforts
- Determine next steps with family
- Recognize that health professionals and families can learn from one another about effective advocacy

Source: Reproduced with permission from Green. M., Palfrey, J.S., Clark, E.M., & Anastasi, J.M. (Eds.) (2002). *Bright futures: Guidelines for health supervision of infants, children, and adolescents* (2nd ed., rev.)—*Pocket guide.* Arlington, VA: National Center for Education in Maternal and Child Health.

Advocacy: Session 1

DEFINING ADVOCACY AND OTHER RELATED TERMS

Advocacy

The act of pleading or arguing in favor of something, such as a cause, an idea, or a policy; active support (*American Heritage Dictionary* definition)

Legislative Terms

Bills • Measures proposing legislation to create a new law or program or amend or repeal existing law

Acts • Bills that have been passed in both houses of Congress

Laws • Acts passed by both houses of Congress and signed by the president, or passed after presidential veto

Authorizations • Legislation to establish a proposed government program

Appropriations • Legislation to provide the money to fund government programs that have already been established by authorizing legislation

Lobbyist • An individual who tries to influence the thinking of legislators or other public officials to either promote or prevent passage of specific legislation

Advocacy: Session 1

STEPWISE: THE FOUR-STEP APPROACH TO ADVOCACY

STEP 1: Identify Family Needs or Concerns

STEP 2: Assess the Situation

STEP 3: Develop a Strategy

STEP 4: Follow Through

Advocacy: Session 1

CASE VIGNETTE:
TAYLOR'S LEARNING PROBLEMS

It has been a busy clinic day, and you have three patients remaining. You pick up the next chart and see that the patient is Taylor, a 9-year-old girl. You quickly review the note from her last visit a year ago. Taylor was doing well in the second grade. Her growth parameters were between the 50th and 75th percentile, and her physical exam was normal. She had a normal hearing and vision screen at the last visit.

You walk into the exam room and greet Taylor and her mother. You begin by reviewing the previous visit and ask, "How is Taylor doing? What questions or concerns do you have at this time?"

Taylor's mother responds, "I don't know what to do. Taylor was doing well in school last year, but this year in third grade she seems to be having more trouble with reading and writing. She is really struggling, and I want to know what I can do to get help for her."

Advocacy: Session 1

SESSION EVALUATION FORM

Session 1: Advocating for the Needs of an Individual

Date: _______________________________

Facilitator(s): _______________________________

Site: _______________________________

1. Overall, I found the "Advocating for the Needs of an Individual" session to be:

Not Useful			Very Useful	
1	2	3	4	5

2. The objectives of the session were:

Not Clear				Clear
1	2	3	4	5

3. The organization of the session was:

Poor				Excellent
1	2	3	4	5

4. The communication skills of the facilitator(s) were:

Poor				Excellent
1	2	3	4	5

5. The facilitator(s) stimulated interest in the subject matter:

Not at All			Very Much	
1	2	3	4	5

6. The facilitator(s) encouraged group participation:

Not at All			Very Much	
1	2	3	4	5

7. Handouts or visual aids (if used) were:

Not Helpful		Very Helpful		
1	2	3	4	5

8. Any additional comments?

____

____

____

9. The most useful features of the session were:

____

____

____

10. Suggestions for improvement

____

____

____

11. Suggestions for topics related to this session

____

____

Advocacy: Session 1

LEARNER SELF-ASSESSMENT FORM

1. Define advocacy.

2. Describe the four-step approach to advocacy.

3. Describe a situation in which you might apply the four-step approach and how you would do it.

4. How will you apply what you have learned in this session to your practice?

Advocacy: Session 1

FACILITATOR SELF-ASSESSMENT FORM

Directions: Please rate yourself from 1 to 5 on the following facilitator skills. The closer you are to a 5 within each domain, the more skilled you are at facilitation. We encourage you to complete this form prior to and after each teaching experience (e.g., a single session or an entire module). This will allow you to assess your performance as a facilitator over time.

Facilitator Behavior	1	2	3	4	5
Remains neutral					
Does not judge ideas					
Keeps the group focused on common task					
Asks clarifying questions					
Creates a climate free of criticism					
Encourages participation					
Structures participation					

Source: Adapted with permission from Welch, M. (1999). *Teaching diversity and cultural competence in health care: A trainer's guide.* San Francisco, CA: Perspectives of Differences Diversity Training and Consultation for Health Professionals (PODSDT).

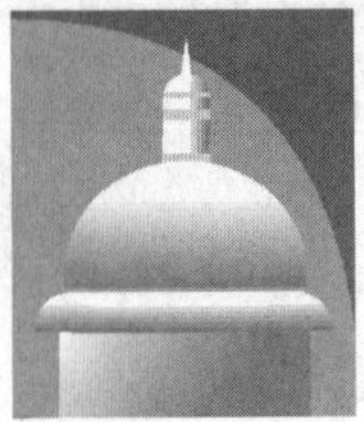

SESSION 2:
Advocating for the Needs of a Group

At the beginning of the session, the facilitator and learners should introduce themselves briefly. (If the same group has recently completed Session 1, the facilitator may decide that introductions are not needed.) Ideas for creative introductions can be found in the Facilitator's Guide.

Setting the Context: The Bright Futures Concept

(May be omitted if recently presented or when sessions are combined.)

The facilitator **(F)** introduces the learners to the Bright Futures concept of health by reading or paraphrasing the following:

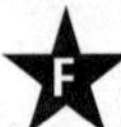 *The World Health Organization has defined health as "a state of complete physical, mental and social well-being and not merely the absence of disease or infirmity." Bright Futures embraces this broad definition of health—one that includes not only prevention of morbidity and mortality, but also the achievement of a child's full potential. In the Bright Futures concept of health, providing the capacity for healthy child development is as important as ameliorating illness or injury. Recognizing and acknowledging the strengths and resources of the child, family, and community are essential to promoting healthy growth and development.*

To build that capacity, the Pediatrics in Practice *curriculum focuses on six core concepts: Partnership, Communication, Health Promotion/Illness Prevention, Time Management, Education, and Advocacy. The curriculum also includes a companion module (Health) and videotape that present an overview of* Pediatrics in Practice *and the Bright Futures approach.*

Introducing the Session

Before introducing the session, the facilitator distributes the handout **Advocacy: Advocating for Children, Families, and Communities** to the learners. (The facilitator may choose not to distribute the handout if it was recently given to the same learners.)

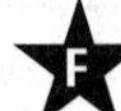 *Today's session is the second of two that comprise the* Pediatrics in Practice *Advocacy module. [Optional: Your* **Advocacy: Advocating for Children, Families, and Communities** *handout outlines the steps involved in advocating for children, families, and communities. We will cover these steps in more detail as we go through today's session.] In the last session, we defined advocacy and applied the four-step approach to advocating for the needs of an individual. Today we will apply the same steps to advocating for the needs of a group.*

In today's session, our objectives will be to:

▶ *Review and reinforce your understanding of the four-step approach to advocacy*

▶ *Practice using the four-step approach to advocate for the needs of a group on the local or national level*

When we have completed the session, you should be able to answer the following question:

▶ *How do I, as a pediatric provider, determine where and how to focus my advocacy efforts?*

Discussion and Exercises

Stepwise: The Four-Step Approach to Advocacy

The facilitator can use the case vignette in this session to focus the discussion on one of two areas:

Option 1: Advocating for Helmet Use in the Community

How to obtain information about helmet use to better educate the community and to advocate for more effective helmet use laws.

or

Option 2: Advocating for Safe Riding Conditions in the Community

How to partner with the boy and his parents to advocate for changes to prevent future injuries and promote a safer environment for the children in the community.

Please note that the introductory discussion for Options 1 and 2 will be identical up to Step 1b, where one area of focus for advocacy is chosen. At that point, the facilitator will continue the discussion of the four-step approach with examples based on helmet use (Option 1, this page) or examples related to safe riding conditions (Option 2, p. 244).

The facilitator distributes the handouts **Stepwise: The Four-Step Approach to Advocacy** and **Case Vignette: John's Emergency Department Visit**.

Option 1: Advocating for Helmet Use in the Community

The facilitator begins as follows:

Would one of you please read the vignette aloud to the group?

Using the display board or flip chart, the facilitator notes the first step in the four-step approach:

STEP 1: Identify Group Needs or Concerns

a. Use open-ended questions to identify specific group needs or concerns

Using open-ended questions, gather more information about conditions for bike riding and helmet use in the community.

Examples:

▶ What concerns do you have about the condition of the parking lot where you ride your bike? Do others share these concerns?

▶ How do your friends try to pressure you to do things that you don't want to do? How do you handle that?

▶ What makes you angry about having to wear a helmet?

▶ How has your town tried to help kids get a space for safe riding?

▶ What thoughts do you have about trying to do something to improve the space where kids rollerblade, skateboard, and ride their bikes?

b. Choose a specific area of focus

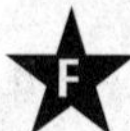
Can you identify some possible areas of advocacy, based on what you have learned so far?

Suggestions can be posted on the display board or on a flip chart. There are several areas of focus that may be identified by the learners, including helmet use and safe riding conditions in the community. The following examples focus on helmet use. If the facilitator chooses to focus on a discussion of advocating for safe riding conditions in the community, see Option 2 on page 244.

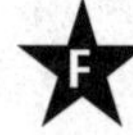
You have identified several possible areas of focus for advocacy in this case. In our discussion today, we are going to use examples based on advocating for helmet use in the community.

Suggestions for advocating for helmet use in the community might include:

▶ Changing the laws regarding helmet use for skating and biking

▶ Developing education programs for children and parents in the town

▶ Coordinating with schools, local police, libraries, and hospital programs on other strategies for educating the community

▶ Educating the children and families in your practice about helmet use

c. Clarify family's beliefs and expectations about the issue

▶ Do John and/or his parents believe that helmet laws could be changed for the better?

▶ What would change John's mind about helmet use?

d. Determine what has been done to date, and what has (or has not) worked

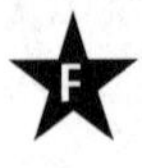 *In response to your questions, you have learned:*

- John is angry about wearing a helmet because some of his friends don't wear helmets. Most did wear helmets when they were "little kids," but many do not now. Many of the teens show up with helmets hanging on their bikes.

- Still, John says he tries to hang around the ones who do wear helmets. He understands why he should wear a helmet, but he would never try to convince his friends to wear one.

- A little while ago, one friend fell off his bike while doing a flip. He didn't have a helmet and required lots of stitches in his head. John says that the boy still doesn't wear his helmet.

e. Do some initial "fact finding" and obtain data

 *In this case, a review of visit histories reveals that other children from the same community have been injured recently. What other "fact finding" might you do?*

- Collect data from sources such as local emergency departments (searching for visits by zip code, for example); local public health departments (searching for injuries by town); or school nurses and local emergency medical services personnel.

f. Talk with others, determine progress to date on the issue

 *Ask others about what resources might be available to you.*

STEP 2: Assess the Situation

a. Determine existing community resources

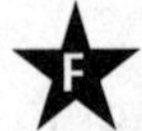 *What other resources are available to you?*

- Are there local bike safety coalitions or injury prevention programs that can assist you?

b. Learn the laws

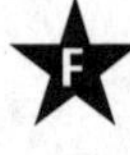 *Is there a law that addresses what you are advocating for?*

- Is there a law that requires bike helmet use (state vs. local ordinance)?

- Was a bill recently introduced and turned down?

- Is there a bill in the legislature that addresses this issue? Does it only cover certain age groups?

c. Review the data and resources

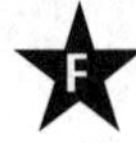 *Review all the information you've gathered. Make sure your efforts will benefit the population at risk. Review the list of possible areas of focus and verify which issues your data best support.*

- In this situation, if you work on changing the law to require helmet use for all children younger than 14 years of age, yet the injuries are occurring in children older than 14, you will not affect the population for which you are advocating.

d. Assess the political or service climate

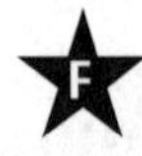 *Is the local political climate right for this issue at this time? Is it of interest to anyone else?*

For example:

- If the community is having problems with head injuries from other sporting activities (e.g., skateboarding, rollerblading, skiing), a focus on helmet use might improve that situation.

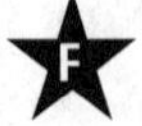 *Also, know your opposition or support. Who or what might oppose or support you in your advocacy efforts?*

- Other groups, such as motorcycle clubs or ski groups, may emerge in opposition to or in support of the helmet use issue. Determine if these groups exist and what they have done in the past to either oppose or support helmet use. Are there opportunities to partner with others to maximize resources?

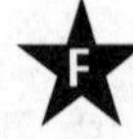 *Once you identify what the opposition would be, try to determine if you can address it.*

- For helmet use, it would be important to recruit the community's public safety officials or police department to support the plan.

STEP 3: Develop a Strategy

a. Limit efforts to a specific issue

In the first session, the advocacy efforts in the case vignette about Taylor's learning problems were limited to issues relating specifically to her needs—getting her a specific needed service. When advocating for the needs of a group, it is important to focus on a single issue, and perhaps even a single strategy within that issue, for maximum impact and the best chance of success.

Let's look at the list of focus areas we developed earlier (listed below).

Which of these areas of focus would you pursue in response to this case vignette about John and his visit to the Emergency Department?

- ▶ Changing the laws
- ▶ Educating children, parents, and the community
- ▶ Looking at what can be done within your own practice

b. Use existing resources

If the learners have chosen one of the three focus areas suggested, start with the existing resources listed below for their chosen area of focus and ask them to suggest other action steps that can be taken. Then briefly go over the suggested existing resources for the other specific issues that were not chosen.

Changing the laws

- ▶ Work with community leaders or the police department to pass a local ordinance that mandates helmet use and restricts skating and riding in areas designated as off-limits to those who do not comply with the ordinance.
- ▶ Work with an injury prevention coalition to change local or state laws to address the issue of helmet use.

Educating kids, parents, and the community

- ▶ Speak to the local police about a positive incentive program for children.
- ▶ Create an educational program in the town to highlight the importance of helmet use.
- ▶ Work with families to begin a program to monitor the kids for helmet use while they are riding in the parking lot.
- ▶ Partner with a local store owner to obtain coupons for free items (e.g., ice cream cone) that community leaders (e.g., police, civic leaders,

store owners) can pass out to children wearing helmets.

- ▶ Hold a bike rodeo. Have the children plan the event as part of a school assignment or other community activity.
- ▶ Enlist the staff from the local Parks and Recreation Department to assist with community-based events.

Looking at what can be done within your own practice

- ▶ Have brochures on safe riding practices (including helmet use) available in your reception areas or examination rooms.
- ▶ Sponsor a safety poster contest for the children in your practice and display the posters.

c. Start with small steps and build upon success

 *Decide what is most "do-able" and has the best chance for success. After an issue is chosen, prioritize your action plan.*

- ▶ Start with what is available (e.g., existing legislation) to address the issue.
- ▶ Work to modify what might be in place but is not quite effective.
- ▶ Work on new approaches or resources.

STEP 4: Follow Through

a. Be passionate about the issue

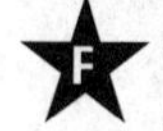 *Commit yourself to the issue or need, but be willing to negotiate.*

b. Review the outcome

 *Keep abreast of and reexamine the different steps in your action plan as you take them.*

c. Evaluate your efforts

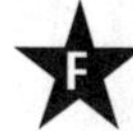 *Reflect on your effort to date. Ask yourself and/or your community partners the following questions:*

- ▶ What worked, what didn't work, and why?
- ▶ What else needs to be done?
- ▶ What data can you gather to evaluate the success of your efforts?

d. Determine next steps in partnership with those you are working with

Attend follow-up meetings, or suggest that a meeting be held to discuss the steps that should be taken to ensure that your efforts are sustained in the community.

> ▶ What might happen as a result of the various strategies you have undertaken?

> ▶ How can the partners communicate and support each other to achieve the action plan?

e. Learn from one another

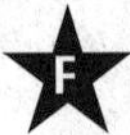 *Advocating at a community level can be time consuming and often frustrating. As a child health professional, however, you should be aware that your voice and participation in advocacy efforts can have a profound impact on policy issues in the community. Partnering with community members provides an opportunity to learn from each other while working on a common, shared interest.*

Option 2: Advocating for Safe Riding Conditions in the Community

The facilitator begins as follows:

 *Would one of you please read the vignette aloud to the group?*

Using the display board or flip chart, the facilitator notes the first step in the four-step approach:

STEP 1: Identify Group Needs or Concerns

a. Use open-ended questions to identify specific group needs or concerns

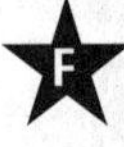 *Using open-ended questions, gather more information about conditions for bike riding and helmet use in the community.*

Examples:

▶ What concerns do you have about the condition of the parking lot where you ride your bike? Do others share these concerns?

▶ How do your friends try to pressure you to do things that you don't want to do? How do you handle that?

▶ What makes you angry about having to wear a helmet?

▶ How has your town tried to help kids get a space for safe riding?

▶ What thoughts do you have about trying to

do something to improve the space where kids rollerblade, skateboard, and ride their bikes?

b. Choose a specific area of focus

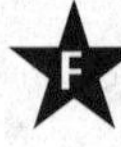 *Can you identify some possible areas of advocacy, based on what you have learned so far?*

Suggestions can be posted on the display board or on a flip chart. There are several areas of focus that may be identified by the learners, including helmet use and safe riding conditions in the community. The following examples focus on advocating for safe riding conditions in the community. If the facilitator chooses to focus on a discussion of advocating for helmet use in the community, see Option 1 on page 241.

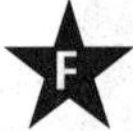 *You have identified several possible areas of focus for advocacy in this case. In our discussion today, we are going to use examples based on advocating for safe riding conditions in the community.*

Suggestions for advocating for a safe riding place for the children in the community might include:

> ▶ Working to improve available skating and biking areas or creating a new one

> ▶ Coordinating with others in the community to identify and promote safe play areas

c. Clarify family's beliefs and expectations about the issue

▶ What concerns do you have about the parking lot?

▶ About places available for safe riding?

d. Determine what has been done to date, and what has (or has not) worked

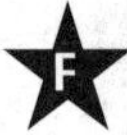 *In response to your questions, you have learned:*

> ▶ The parking lot is in bad condition. It's in an old industrial area, but it is the only open lot where children can ride and not be bothered.

> ▶ John and his friends complain among themselves and have tried to ride in some other business parking lots, but they have been chased away or asked to leave.

> ▶ John and his friends try to be "cool" by taking chances on their bikes and

skateboards, doing flips and spins. There is pressure to do this, to be part of the "in" group.

- Different groups of teens use the lot. There's a real tough group, but John says he doesn't like to hang around them. He avoids the lot when he sees that this group is there.
- John says that all the teens would love to have a skate park. Once in a while, they get to go to other towns that have them, but no one is doing anything about creating one in their community.
- John and his friends once tried to clean things up, but they feel that no one cares. Most of the debris is too big for them to move. There's glass and dirt and they have nowhere to put it.

e. Do some initial "fact-finding" and obtain data

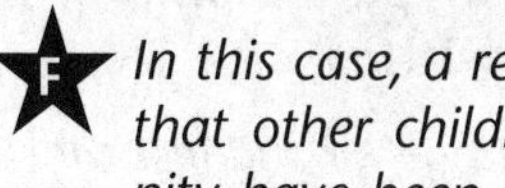 *In this case, a review of visit histories reveals that other children from the same community have been injured recently. What other "fact-finding" might you do?*

- Contact the local police or town government officials to determine if any efforts have been made in the past or are currently under way to improve the conditions where the children ride.

f. Talk with others, determine progress to date on the issue

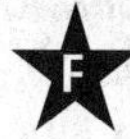 *Ask others about what resources might be available to you.*

STEP 2: Assess the Situation

a. Determine existing community resources

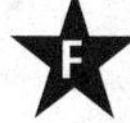 *What other resources are available to you?*

- Are there local bike safety coalitions or injury prevention programs that can assist you?

b. Learn the laws

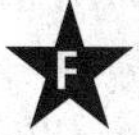 *Is there a law that addresses what you are advocating for?*

- Is there a local ordinance that applies to the use of parking lots for recreational use?

c. Review the data

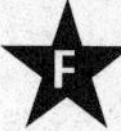 *Review all the information you've gathered. Make sure your efforts will benefit the population at risk. Review the list of possible areas of focus and verify which issues your data best support.*

- If you focus on safe places for bike riding, but the injuries are occurring to children on rollerblades and skateboards, you will miss the intended population.

d. Assess the political or service climate

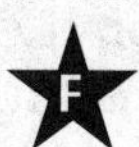 *Is the local political climate right for this issue at this time? Is it of interest to anyone else?*

For example:

- If the community is having problems with teen mischief and vandalism, your suggestion for a supervised, teen-focused activity area might improve that situation.

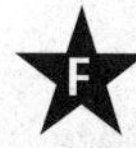 *Also, know your opposition or support. Who or what might oppose you in your advocacy efforts?*

- In this case, location could be a key issue. The elderly or busy business merchants who favor passive recreation areas would probably have a concern about creating a safe area for skating or biking.

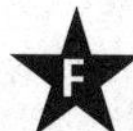 *Once you identify what the opposition would be, try to determine if you can address it.*

- For this issue, it would be important to recruit the community's public safety officials or police department to support the plan.

STEP 3: Develop a Strategy

a. Limit efforts to a specific issue

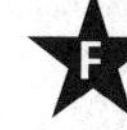 *In the first session, the advocacy efforts in the case vignette about Taylor's learning problems were limited to issues relating specifically to her needs—getting her a specific needed service. When advocating for the needs of a group, it is important to focus on a single issue, and perhaps even a single strategy within that issue, for maximum impact and the best chance of success.*

Let's look at the list of focus areas we developed earlier (listed below).

Which of these areas of focus would you pursue in response to this case vignette about

John and his visit to the Emergency Department?

- ▶ Changing the laws
- ▶ Improving access to safe riding and skating spaces for children
- ▶ Educating children, parents, and the community
- ▶ Looking at what can be done within your own practice

b. Use existing resources

If the learners have chosen one of the four focus areas suggested, start with the existing resources listed below for their chosen area of focus and ask them to suggest other action steps that can be taken. Then briefly go over the suggested existing resources for the other specific issues that were not chosen.

Changing the laws

- ▶ Work with community leaders or the police department to pass a local ordinance that restricts skating and riding in designated areas.

Improving access to safe riding and skating spaces for children

- ▶ Work with the children and their families to explore the possibility of creating a park.
- ▶ Work with the children and their families to raise funds to clean and repave the lot.
- ▶ Recruit and work with other groups in different communities who have addressed the same issue with some success.

Educating kids, parents, and the community

- ▶ Speak to the local police about a positive incentive program for children.
- ▶ Work with parents to begin a program to monitor the kids in the parking lot.

c. Start with small steps and build upon success

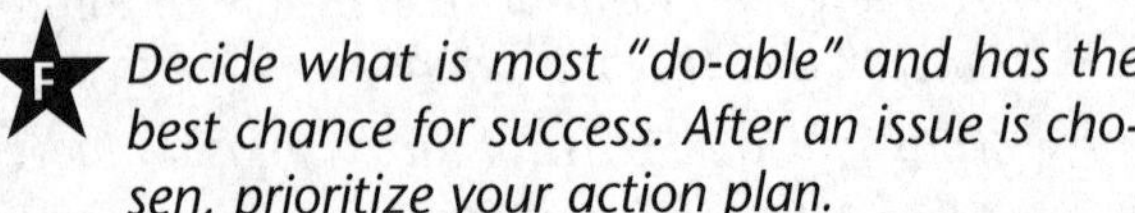 *Decide what is most "do-able" and has the best chance for success. After an issue is chosen, prioritize your action plan.*

- ▶ Start with what is available (e.g., existing legislation) to address the issue.

- ▶ Work to modify what might be in place but is not quite appropriate.
- ▶ Work on new approaches or resources.

STEP 4: Follow Through

a. Be passionate about the issue

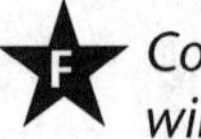 *Commit yourself to the issue or need, but be willing to negotiate*

b. Review the outcome

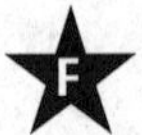 *Keep abreast of and reexamine the different steps in your action plan as you take them.*

c. Evaluate your efforts

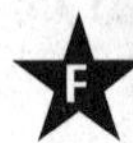 *Reflect on your effort to date. Ask yourself and/or your community partners the following questions:*

- ▶ What worked, what didn't work, and why?
- ▶ What else needs to be done?

d. Determine next steps in partnership with those you are working with

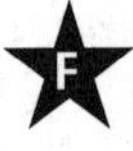 *Attend follow-up meetings, or suggest that a meeting be held to discuss the steps that should be taken to ensure that your efforts are sustained in the community.*

e. Learn from one another

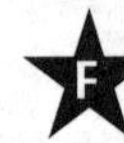 *Advocating at a community level can be time consuming and often frustrating. As a child health professional, however, you should be aware that your voice and participation in advocacy efforts can have a profound impact on policy issues in the community. Partnering with community members provides an opportunity to learn from each other while working on a common, shared interest.*

Take-Home Message

The facilitator ends the session with the following:

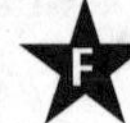 *In this session, you have applied the four-step advocacy process at the community level. Working in collaboration with other groups in the community is essential for moving the issue forward, reducing duplicate efforts, and developing a common, shared voice. Child health professionals are important partners in recognizing, developing, and supporting policies that affect children's health. Before*

we conclude, what questions remain about what we addressed today?

Answer to the Guiding Question

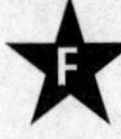 *Now that we have completed this session on Advocacy, you should be able to answer the following question:*

▶ How do I, as a pediatric provider, determine where and how to focus my advocacy efforts?

- After eliciting child and family concerns, the pediatric provider should assess the situation to gather facts, document the problem, and gauge the political climate.

Evaluation

The facilitator now distributes the **Session Evaluation Form** and the **Learner Self-Assessment Form.** The facilitator also completes the **Facilitator Self-Assessment Form.**

Advocacy: Session 2

ADVOCACY: ADVOCATING FOR CHILDREN, FAMILIES, AND COMMUNITIES

Health professionals can be involved in advocacy either at an individual level (for example, obtaining services for a child or family) or at a local or national level (speaking with the media, community groups, or legislators).

1. Identify Family Needs or Concerns.
- Use open-ended questions to identify specific needs or concerns of the family
  Example: "What are some of the main concerns in your life right now?"
- Choose a specific area of focus
  Example: Obtaining special education services for a child.
- Clarify family's beliefs and expectations about the issue
- Determine what has been done to date, and what has (or hasn't) worked
  Example: Parents may have tried unsuccessfully to obtain services for their child.
- Do some initial "fact finding" and obtain data
  Example: Contact board of education or local department of public health.
- Talk with others, determine progress
  Example: Is there a local school coalition that addresses the issue?

2. Assess the Situation.
- Determine existing community resources
- Learn the laws
  Example: Are there any existing laws that address the issue?
- Review the data and resources to be sure they support the issue
- Assess political climate to determine support or opposition
  Example: Is this issue of interest to anyone else (school/early intervention teacher, local policymakers)? Who (or what) might oppose the advocacy efforts? Why?

3. Develop a Strategy.
- Limit efforts to a specific issue
  Example: Obtaining special education services for a child rather than changing the laws.
- Use existing resources
- Start with small steps, then build upon successes
  Examples: Write a letter to the school district. Attend the special education evaluation.

4. Follow Through.
- Be passionate about the issue, but willing to negotiate
- Review the outcome
- Evaluate your efforts
- Determine next steps with family
- Recognize that health professionals and families can learn from one another about effective advocacy

Source: Reproduced with permission from Green. M., Palfrey, J.S., Clark, E.M., & Anastasi, J.M. (Eds.) (2002). *Bright futures: Guidelines for health supervision of infants, children, and adolescents* (2nd ed., rev.)—*Pocket guide.* Arlington, VA: National Center for Education in Maternal and Child Health.

Advocacy: Session 2

STEPWISE: THE FOUR-STEP APPROACH TO ADVOCACY

STEP 1: Identify Family Needs or Concerns

STEP 2: Assess the Situation

STEP 3: Develop a Strategy

STEP 4: Follow Through

Advocacy: Session 2

CASE VIGNETTE:
JOHN'S EMERGENCY DEPARTMENT VISIT

One evening while working in the Emergency Department (ED) you care for a 14-year-old boy, John, who sustained a facial laceration while performing tricks on his bike at a parking lot in his town. He was wearing a helmet at the time. He tells you he is angry that he has to wear a helmet but says that his mother insists on it. The nurse attending to John comments that he is the third child this week who has visited the ED with an injury. She believes they all were injured in the same place. This information piques your curiosity. While you are waiting for a consultation on John's injuries, you look up the visit histories on the previous two cases. You discover that they did in fact occur at the same location.

Advocacy: Session 2

SESSION EVALUATION FORM

Session 2: Advocating for the Needs of a Group

Date: _________________________

Facilitator(s): _________________________

Site: _________________________

---

1. Overall, I found the "Advocating for the Needs of a Group" session to be:

Not Useful				Very Useful
1	2	3	4	5

2. The objectives of the session were:

Not Clear				Clear
1	2	3	4	5

3. The organization of the session was:

Poor				Excellent
1	2	3	4	5

4. The communication skills of the facilitator(s) were:

Poor				Excellent
1	2	3	4	5

5. The facilitator(s) stimulated interest in the subject matter:

Not at All				Very Much
1	2	3	4	5

6. The facilitator(s) encouraged group participation:

Not at All				Very Much
1	2	3	4	5

7. Handouts or visual aids (if used) were:

Not Helpful				Very Helpful
1	2	3	4	5

8. Any additional comments?

   ____

   ____

   ____

9. The most useful features of the session were:

   ____

   ____

   ____

10. Suggestions for improvement

    ____

    ____

    ____

11. Suggestions for topics related to this session

    ____

    ____

    ____

Advocacy: Session 2

LEARNER SELF-ASSESSMENT FORM

1. Describe the four-step approach to advocacy.

2. Describe a situation in a community where you might apply the four-step approach. Briefly describe how you would do it.

3. How will you apply what you have learned in this session to your practice?

Advocacy: Session 2

FACILITATOR SELF-ASSESSMENT FORM

Directions: Please rate yourself from 1 to 5 on the following facilitator skills. The closer you are to a 5 within each domain, the more skilled you are at facilitation. We encourage you to complete this form prior to and after each teaching experience (e.g., a single session or an entire module). This will allow you to assess your performance as a facilitator over time.

Facilitator Behavior	1	2	3	4	5
Remains neutral					
Does not judge ideas					
Keeps the group focused on common task					
Asks clarifying questions					
Creates a climate free of criticism					
Encourages participation					
Structures participation					

Source: Adapted with permission from Welch, M. (1999). *Teaching diversity and cultural competence in health care: A trainer's guide.* San Francisco, CA: Perspectives of Differences Diversity Training and Consultation for Health Professionals (PODSDT).

References

Benjamin, J.T., Cimino, S.A., & Hafler, J.P., Bright Futures Health Promotion Work Group, & Bernstein, H.H. (2002). The office visit: A time to promote health—but how? *Contemporary Pediatrics, 19*(2), 90–107.

Berman, S. (1998). Training pediatricians to become child advocates. *Pediatrics, 102*(3), 632–636.

Dolins, J.C., & Christoffel, K.K. (1994). Reducing violent injuries: Priorities for pediatrician advocacy. *Pediatrics, 94*(4 Part 2), 638–651.

Durkin, M.S., Laraque, D., Lubman, I., Barlow, B. (1999). Epidemiology and prevention of traffic injuries to urban children and adolescents. *Pediatrics, 103*(6), e74.

Green, M., & Palfrey, J.S., (Eds.) (2002). *Bright futures: Guidelines for gealth supervision of infants, children, and adolescents* (2nd ed., rev.). Arlington, VA: National Center for Education in Maternal and Child Health.

Green, M., Palfrey, J.S., Clark, E.M., & Anastasi, J.M., (Eds.) (2002). *Bright futures: Guidelines for gealth supervision of infants, children, and adolescents* (2nd ed., rev.)—*Pocket guide.* Arlington, VA: National Center for Education in Maternal and Child Health.

Knitzer, J. (1976_. Child advocacy: A perspective. *American Journal of Orthopsychiatry, 46*(2), 200–216.

Laraque, D., Barlow, B., Davidson, L., & Welborn, C. (1994). Central Harlem Playground Injury Prevention Project: A model for change. *American Journal of Public Health, 84*(10), 1691–1692.

Laraque, D., Barlow, B., Durkin, M., & Heagarty, M. (1995). Injury prevention in an urban setting: Challenges and successes. *Journal of Urban Health: Bulletin of the New York Academy of Medicine, 72*(1), 16–30.

Laraque, D., Spivak, H., & Bull, M. (2001). Serious firearm injury prevention does make sense. *Pediatrics, 107*(2), 408–411.

Lozano, P., Biggs, V.M., Sibley, B.J., Smith, T.M., Marcuse, E.K., & Bergman, A.B. (1994). Advocacy training during pediatric residency. *Pediatrics, 94*(4), 532–536.

Sege, R., & Dietz, W. (1994). Television viewing and violence in children: The pediatrician as agent for change. *Pediatrics, 94*(4), 600–607.

Wilson-Brewer, R., & Spivak, H. (1994). Violence prevention in schools and other community settings: The pediatrician as initiator, educator, collaborator, and advocate. *Pediatrics, 94*(4), 623–630.

Resources

AAP, State Government Affairs: www.aap.org.

Injury Free Coalition for Kids: www.injuryfree.org.

PAX, the movement to end gun violence: www.AskingSavesKids.com.

Wallack, L., Dorfman, L., Jernigan, D., & Themba, M. (1993). *Media advocacy and public health: Power for Prevention.* Thousands Oaks, CA: Sage Publications, Inc.

INDEX